# Let's Talk
# Dementia
## A Caregiver's Guide

Carol Howell

This is a well written book for the families affected by Alzheimer's disease. It is easy to understand and provides excellent education and guidance to the caregivers in their struggle to manage their relatives. This should be a must read for anyone involved in Alzheimer's care.

*M. Reza Bolouri, MD*

"Spot on advice from someone who knows dementia. If someone you love has dementia, you need this book."

*Dr. Steve Oehme*

# Acknowledgements

The journey of dementia can be scary, confusing, and frustrating. It can also be meaningful, filled with love, and laced with humor. I know this first hand. My life is filled with individuals God has placed in my life who allow me to experience all these emotions. Most of all, I am blessed to be one of the caregivers for my wonderful Momma. Vera Jean Holder entered this world in the mountains of North Carolina, married and moved to New Mexico at the ripe age of 15, and started her family a few years later.

I am the second of three daughters, and I have always been proud to be Vera's daughter. Momma has always exemplified the qualities of a good wife, mother, friend, and Child of God. She has the heart and spirit I want to portray to all whom I am blessed to meet as we, together, travel this journey of dementia.

"Momma, I love you too much for words. There will never be a day I don't treasure our moments together. Thank you for loving me more than I love myself. Thank you for helping me to see something in me that only a mother could recognize. Thank you for loving our Lord and teaching me about Him. Thank you for being YOU. I couldn't ask for any more."

Carol

# MY STORY

"Hello, Mrs. Howell. This is Dr. Wrong. I am calling to let you know your mother has dementia." Shocked, I responded, "Are you calling to tell me my mother might *get* dementia?" "No m'am. She *has* dementia. I will call in a prescription for her. Let me know if you need anything," he responded. I sat on the edge of the bed in a state of bewilderment and said to my husband, "I'm either going to pass out or throw-up. I don't know which."

That Thursday morning, August 2006, my world changed. I will never forget that day. However, knowing what I do now about Alzheimer's, I can't be sure of that last statement. Alzheimer's and dementia have long played a part in my world. My grandmother, Bessie, was diagnosed with dementia many years ago. For a long time Grandma would say, "I just don't feel right". None of us really knew what that meant, but Grandma was aware of a change going on in her body. It was many years later before her diagnosis was made. She battled this disease of Alzheimer's like the trooper she always was, but it finally claimed her life. I have some wonderful stories about Grandma, and I can't wait to share them with you.

When Momma's diagnosis entered my world, my first thoughts were those of Grandma and what her life was like during her last few months. I was scared. My Aunt Evelyn cared for Grandma in her home. She had the sole responsibility for Grandma's every need. I knew this would be my job for Momma. I was more than happy to accept this responsibility, but I was more than a little bit frightened. After all, I had just been told my Mother had a fatal disease, and this information was given to me over the phone! What kind of doctor does this? There were no warm, fuzzy, understanding emotions tied to the announcement. Only cold facts.

I began doing what lots of females do in times of struggle. I participated in "shower cries". I will bet you are familiar with "shower cries". That is when you cry in the shower for as long as you like. It works because no one knows you are crying. When you get out of the shower, and your face is all red from the crying, you blame it on the hot shower water. It worked wonderfully…for a short while. Then reality set in, and I knew I must learn everything I could about dementia and Alzheimer's. But, wait a minute. Dr. Wrong never said my Momma had Alzheimer's. Ahh, I felt so much better once this realization hit!

The internet and I became best friends. That is where I learned the definition of "dementia", and simply put, it is the inability to think clearly. I was good with that definition. It certainly described what I was seeing in my Momma.

At the time of her diagnosis, Momma was working at a local furniture store. She consistently was among the top salespeople each month. I am not wrong when I say, "Momma could sell ice to an Eskimo and sunshine to a Floridian". She had that certain something that made you want to talk to her, listen to her, and pull out your credit card to buy from her. Momma previously owned a La-Z-Boy Showcase Shoppe in Fayetteville, North Carolina. She worked in and managed this store like the professional she was. You would have thought she graduated from a school of business, but she graduated from the "school of hard knocks", instead. Prior to her La-Z-Boy days, Momma made appointments for Mr. Faulkner to test the hearing of individuals in their home. Mr. Faulkner had it made! My Momma had already sold these people on their need for a hearing aid long before he ever stepped foot in their door.

After the La-Z-Boy experience, Momma sold jewelry. I might have had a nice inheritance in my future if Momma had never entered that jewelry store. It seemed the more she sold – and she sold a great deal – the more she purchased. She came home once with a ring I called her "big butt" ring and announced the purchase price of said ring. Considering she purchased this ring at cost, I just about fainted. Not only did it cost almost as much as the first house I purchased in 1980, it was UGLY! Not just a little bit ugly. No, it was really ugly! Looking back on this, I can't blame this purchase on the dementia. Momma really liked this ring. Go figure!

However, Momma began having problems at work. It seemed she had not lost her knack to sell, but her ability to complete the paperwork was becoming quite an issue. She had asked her employer if the office could handle the paperwork end of her job  thus giving her time to concentrate on sales. While this seemed like a logical solution, it was not fair to the other employees. As a result, Momma muddled her way through the business end of each sale. When mistakes in math started popping up, directions to homes for delivery were poorly described, and product numbers transposed, her employer became increasingly concerned.

On the home side of things, one particular day comes to mind. I had been helping Momma manage her assets for quite a few years. While visiting Momma, I noticed three envelopes from the credit union with which she banked. After asking her if I could look at these pieces of mail, I was shocked to learn my Momma had three checks returned for insufficient funds. WHAT? Momma, who had balanced her checkbook without the aid of a calculator her entire life, had bounced three checks? How in the world did this happen? When I asked her, she was totally confused, very upset, and tearful. I offered to help pay her bills. She was happy for the assistance, and this new procedure was put in place.

So, life was changing for Momma. My first goal, since this diagnosis of dementia had entered our world, was to get Momma back to work. Momma needed to work for her own enjoyment and self-edification, and I needed her to work so we could go out to eat! You know, a girl has to look out for her future! I became really excited when I learned there was a difference between dementia and Alzheimer's, and there was something called "reversible dementia". Oh hallelujah!

Before we go further, let me enlighten you. I am a woman of faith. I am proud to say I am a Child of God, and I don't mind sharing my stories of His goodness. When the words "reversible dementia" appeared on my computer screen, I began to pray.

If dementia is "the inability to think clearly", what is Alzheimer's? In my world, and I would guess in most people's, the two were pretty much synonymous. They are not. There are over ninety different reasons a person might have dementia, and Alzheimer's is just one of those reasons. Yes, ninety. I was shocked to learn this bit of information. So what is Alzheimer's then? In simple terms, Alzheimer's is a disease of the brain. We will add to that definition later, but this definition works great for the moment.

Because of Momma's diagnosis, I began investigating this business of reversible and irreversible dementia and gave special attention to the reversible dementias. Momma was still working and being productive. She drove everywhere she needed to go, lived alone, and even cooked her own food. (I will spare you the details of the cabbage with pineapple dish she prepared one night. YUCK!!!)

As I studied, I learned there are several reasons an individual might have a reversible dementia. I began to get excited, and I began to pray. "Please, Lord, let my Momma have one of these reversible dementias. We will get her to the doctor, get the situation corrected, and get her back to work." The reversible dementia I thought most likely in Momma's case, was a reaction to medication. Momma had been suffering from back pain for many months. Because of this pain, she was taking some pretty heavy duty pain medications. In fact, the two of us had almost come to blows when I refused to take her for anymore injections in her spine since they never brought her relief. She became very upset with me. Her state of confusion was becoming increasingly more evident.

During this time of receiving treatment and taking medications for her back pain, Momma took her three daughters on our annual "Girl's Trip". Since you have not had the privilege of going on one of these trips, you will have to take my word when I say, "they were fantastic". Momma paid for everything, and gave all three of us girls a nice little stash of cash with which to shop. The four of us would occupy one dressing room for hours at a time. The trips were so much fun. We laughed, ate, slept, shopped, giggled, told stories, and might have told a few lies. We had a blast.

During our last ever "Girl's Trip" to Myrtle Beach, South Carolina, all three of us noticed how confused Momma had become. She asked the same questions repeatedly, forgot our plans for the day, and became frustrated with herself. We mistakenly wrote these moments off because she was on pain medication.

When I learned medication can be the cause of dementia, I became very excited. I also learned a vitamin B-12 deficiency could cause *sudden onset* dementia. I planned to get Momma's B-12 levels checked immediately. There are several other reasons an individual might exhibit symptoms of dementia, but we will go into those later. For me, I was fixated on this drug reaction and vitamin B-12 deficiency situation.

Straight to the family doctor we went. After explaining about my in-depth research (aka the internet), I asked for a complete blood panel and a discussion about the medications Momma was taking. This doctor, we shall call him Dr. Good, was kind and began to educate us about both dementia and Alzheimer's. He felt sure what Momma had was Alzheimer's, but he was willing to help me see these two trains of thought to their rightful conclusion.

As it turned out, Momma was diagnosed by Dr. Good with Alzheimer's. Alzheimer's is the most common type of dementia. Believe me when I say, "I was not ready for this news". I had prayed for a different outcome, yet it was during this time I was reminded of an important fact. God knows the future. God loves me AND my Momma more than I can ever begin to imagine, and He was not leaving us to fight Alzheimer's alone. He would be our guide, and He had big plans for my life. Alzheimer's had moved in, was a part of the family, and I needed to welcome its presence.

Welcome its presence? Yes! When asked once if I would rather my Mother have Alzheimer's or cancer, I quickly responded, Alzheimer's. What about Alzheimer's or heart disease? Alzheimer's, of course. Why? My Momma is not in pain. Her back problem was corrected with good chiropractic care and a pair of shoes. She has memory issues to deal with, for sure. But Momma is happy. Though I do not look forward to the day she may not recognize me, be in control of her bodily functions, or her body might cease to function because of damage to her brain, she is not suffering. Alzheimer's is not my friend, but I will not fight it. I will learn about it, I will educate about it, and I am determined to help my Momma LIVE with it. My goal in writing this book is to provide you with hands-on tips that will aid you in the day-to-day journey of LIVING with Alzheimer's.

Years have passed since Momma's diagnosis, and life has most certainly changed. Momma decided to move to an assisted living facility. She made this decision on her own, and then announced I would have to figure out how to pay for it all. THANKS, MOMMA! Her memory has slipped a bit more, but she is still a vibrant woman who pretty much runs things at her new home. When her and Pops (her table partner) decide they want to do something, the wonderful employees gather a group of residents and off they go. If Momma wants something special for dinner, they fix it for her. If Momma wants..... and on and on it goes. It's hard to turn this woman down!

As Momma's disease has progressed, I have studied and learned, thought and pondered. I became a Certified Dementia Specialist and an Endorsed Life Coach with an emphasis on dementia. Senior Life Journeys was formed in

2011, and I am proud to speak to groups about dementia as well as coach families through their journey. I also present music therapy to my friends with dementia. It is absolutely the most rewarding part of each week.

My motto is: "Knowledge brings POWER. Power brings HOPE. Hopes brings SMILES." If you are reading this book, you most likely need a smile or two or three. Keep reading. A lot of needed information follows, but I have scattered a few smiles throughout. I love to make my friends with dementia smile.

Smile #1

My brother and I went to the store to purchase ice cream for our dad who was hospitalized. Realizing we would need to purchase spoons, my brother announced he would go back in the store, purchase the spoons, and make a quick stop by the bathroom. It seemed he was gone too long, and I assumed he was having a difficult time finding the plastic spoons. I decided to call him. Little did I know he was in the bathroom when I asked, "Hi, did you have any luck?"

Sometimes, you've just got to laugh!

# WHAT IS DEMENTIA?

I want my words to be easy to understand, and the explanations I give will always follow that format. So, don't be offended at their simplicity. This book is intentionally short, sweet, funny, and to the point.

**Dementia is the inability to think clearly which leads to difficulties with the activities of daily living.**

What are the activities of daily living?

I remember them by the acronym BEAD-T.

- Bathing
- Eating
- Ambulating
- Dressing
- Toileting

For Momma, eating became – and still is – a problem. Momma would skip meals, or she would think she had eaten when she had not actually done so. For many people, the first signs of a problem will arise when they wear the same clothing for several days in a row. Maybe they forget to bathe and odor becomes an issue. These issues should ring a bell in the mind of a loved one.

In addition to problems with memory, dementia may cause a problem with a person's ability to communicate. The thoughts may be in the mind, but the words won't come to the lips. This leads to frustration and even a pulling away from the world in which they normally would participate. It is also common to see a change in a person's reasoning and judgment. We will discuss this more when we learn about the parts of the brain, but dementia is often characterized by a person's lack of inhibitions. As a result, it is not uncommon to hear an individual use words they never would have normally used. This is a warning sign!

Dementia is caused by damage to brain cells that begin to destroy the ability of these cells to communicate with each other. This damage is manifested in the life of the individual based on the particular area of the brain in which the damage occurs. With Alzheimer's, the damage first begins in the hippocampus. The hippocampus is the part of the brain where new memories are made. The damage to this part of the brain makes it difficult, and eventually impossible, for the person to remember new information.

As we learned earlier, dementia can have over ninety different origins. *Alzheimer's is the most common type of dementia*. The second most common type of dementia is called "vascular dementia". This is dementia brought on by a stroke. This dementia may be accompanied by an inability to process language. This happens because the stroke affected the region of the brain that processes language. In this situation, the individual often becomes very frustrated trying to communicate their needs and wants.

Dementia can be caused by Huntington's Disease, Parkinson's Disease, Lewy Body's Disease, Pick's Disease, AIDS, Mad Cow Disease, just to name a few. All of these diseases lead to dementia that is **irreversible**. The number of people with *Alzheimer's dementia* far outweighs all the other dementias. The way the disease affects the body can alter the way the dementia manifests itself with the individual. However, the techniques discussed in this book will be beneficial to anyone caring for a dementia patient no matter their diagnosis.

The main goal of this book is to teach effective ways to make life better for the caregiver and the person with dementia. In addition, it is my desire to reintroduce joy into your life and give you permission to allow humor to take up residence.

The more I learn about dementia, the more I am reminded of the "All I Really Need To Know I Learned In Kindergarten" posters I use to see posted in school rooms. I like to keep those points in mind when caring for someone with dementia.

1. Just because something belongs to you does not mean I might not benefit from using the item.

2. You must always play fair, but I do not. HA HA!

3. It is not uncommon for me to begin hitting people. Don't be shocked if it happens, and please don't yell at me. It is not ME doing the hitting. The disease causes me to do things I would never normally consider doing.

4. It is important you not rearrange my personal belongings. Life is confusing for me. If you move things around, I will be even more confused and unhappy.

5.   Clean up my messes.

6.   I might take things that aren't mine. Don't get upset and accuse me of being a thief. Just quietly remove the item when I am not looking, and return it to its rightful owner. You don't need to discuss it with me. I am not going to remember having taken. However, don't be surprised if I retrieve the item tomorrow.

7.   Please remember to say, "I'm sorry". I still have feelings.

8.   Please wash my hands before I eat.

9.   Remind me to flush.

10.  Cookies and milk help me sleep, but apples and applesauce will keep me awake. Did you know that?

11.  I like to sing, dance, draw, recite poetry, and pray. The side of my brain that holds these activities is least effected by my disease.

12.  I love naps.

13.  Please make sure you hold my hand when we are together. I can get distracted easily, wander off without meaning to do so, and become frightened at the most unusual things. Keep close by, and I will feel safe.

14.  I love flowers, trees, gardens, and nature.

15.  I know my body is changing. I don't understand it, but I am trying my best to deal with it all. Be patient with me, please.

16.  Please pay attention to my non-verbal cues. Sometimes I don't feel good, and I don't have the words to tell you. Sometimes I am tired, and I just need a rest. Sometimes I am hungry, but expressing that is difficult. Please LOOK at my

body and see what you might learn from my non-verbal cues.

Smile #2 -

James and Jane lived on a golf course. Jane took golf lessons from the golf club pro. After the final lesson, the pro told Jane, "Take two weeks off and then quit". James thought it was funny. Jane was not amused.

Sometimes, you've just got to laugh!

# WHAT IS ALZHEIMER'S?

For ease of understanding, the simplest definition is: Alzheimer's is a disease of the brain. If you remember it in those terms, you will be more informed than 99% of the folks you come in contact with.

I could spend some time telling you about beta-amyloid plaque, tau, neurofibrillary tangles, neurons, etc., etc. However, let's keep things simple and easy to remember.

What happens to the brain when Alzheimer's has been diagnosed? Our brain is similar in appearance to a head of cauliflower. It has tight fitting pieces, folds, craters, and sections. The folds in the brain allow for more surface area. In fact, if the average brain were stretched out flat, it would cover an area between 20x11 inches and 20x23 inches in size. That is a lot of brain tissue used to retain the information we need to operate in our world.

The average weight of a human brain is 3 pounds. The female brain is usually smaller than a male brain. Before the men begin thinking too highly of themselves here, let me explain a possible reason for this fact. The female brain's craters and folds are much deeper than the male brain. Therefore, the female brain is just more tightly packed.

When Alzheimer's begins, the first area it likes

to attack is the HIPPOCAMPUS. The hippocampus is located in the medial temporal lobe. OK, let's make that simpler to remember. The temporal lobe is that area just above your ears. In many people, it is the location they most frequently experience headaches. If you were to drill a hole from one side of the head to the other, with the temporal lobe being your beginning point on the left and ending point on the right side of the head, the midway point would be about the location of the hippocampus.

The hippocampus is responsible for our ability to retain new information. Everything you have read thus far is finding a temporary home in your hippocampus. Think of it as a cardboard file box. This file box is a temporary storage place until we decide what to do with the files it contains. Thus, the hippocampus is a temporary storage facility until the information is distributed to another part of the brain to reside in a permanent file box.

When Alzheimer's enters the picture, the hippocampus is damaged and no longer able to retain new information. It shrinks, and cannot hold on to new memories. Further, the memories cannot travel from the temporary file box of the hippocampus to a permanent file box somewhere else in the brain.

Let's look at how this plays out in everyday life.

CAROL – "Momma, you have an appointment at 2PM today to see the cardiologist."

MOMMA – "OK."

A few minutes later....

MOMMA – "What did you say we are doing

today?"

CAROL – "We are going to see the cardiologist at 2PM today."

MOMMA – "Oh yeah. Now I remember. I'm glad I have you to keep me straight!"

CAROL – "I'm glad I have you, too!"

MOMMA – "So, are we doing anything important today?"

As hard as she may try, Momma is not going to remember this new information. Her hippocampus is damaged, and she is physically incapable of retaining the news of an appointment at 2PM.

As the disease progresses, the brain actually begins to deteriorate, and holes develop. Picture the cauliflower again. Now mentally take a knife and drill a hole into that cauliflower. That is much like what happens to the brain with dementia. These holes cause a world of problems for the individual with Alzheimer's.

Our memories, knowledge, intellect, likes, dislikes, bodily commands, etc., are housed within our brain. When holes develop in our brain, these things leave us. The information that was stored in that part of the brain is gone forever. This would explain why Alzheimer's patients forget loved ones, events, appointments, education, and on and on.

This information can be distressing. It is time for another *smile*.

Smile #3

Mary Sue, and her best friend, Ida Bell, (you gotta love those southern names) both widows, had a standing "Girls Night Out" every Friday in their quaint little town in South Carolina. One particular Friday, about 5:30, they drove to the take out window and ordered their meals at Kentucky Fried Chicken, or so they thought. The lady over the speaker replied, "Excuse me, what did you say?" Grace proceeded to order again and the lady then replied, "Grace, honey, (that is what they call each other in these little towns) you are at the bank. The KFC is next door!" Today Grace is 95 years old, living in a home for elders, and she still laughs about that incident.

Sometimes, you've just got to laugh!

# HOW ARE ALZHEIMER'S AND DEMENTIA DIAGNOSED?

I want to look at both Alzheimer's and dementia together when we talk about diagnosing an individual. The first piece of advice anyone should give someone concerned about their loved one is this – GO TO THE DOCTOR! There is no good reason to delay, and every reason to quickly make this appointment.

As I told you earlier, Momma was diagnosed in August of 2006. She had become very confused, agitated, tired, and generally "not with it". I immediately sought a doctor's appointment, and the process of diagnosing began. Looking back on things from an educated view, it is easy to see Momma had dementia. She certainly had an "inability to think clearly", and she was finding life to be more difficult as the days progressed. Our family doctor performed a series of simple questions. "What is the year, date, season? In what state do you live? Who is the President? Count backwards from 100 by increments of seven." Momma had a few problems with the counting backwards part, but I found it rather difficult myself.

One question Momma answered incorrectly seemed totally logical to her. "What doesn't belong in this set of words – sofa, chair, red?" To which Momma didn't have an answer. They all belonged together. You see, Momma had been in the furniture industry for many years. Thinking of sofas and chairs came quite naturally. And, guess what! They both came in red! Putting sofa, chair, and red together made total sense to her. I think that is funny.

Diagnosing Momma's condition began with an evaluation by her family doctor, who then referred her to a neuropsychologist. This doctor administered a battery of tests, and he confirmed her diagnosis of dementia. The diagnosis of Alzheimer's was made in two manners. He ruled out all the reasons Momma might have dementia, and the conclusion remained Alzheimer's. Remember, Alzheimer's is the most common type of dementia. We were also asked, "What was the first symptom of dementia your Mother displayed?" The answer was "loss of short term memory". This is consistent with a diagnosis of Alzheimer's.

If an individual is diagnosed with dementia caused by Parkinson's disease, for example, the first symptom of a problem with the individual may have been tremors. These tremors may have progressed to include other symptoms of Parkinson's, and dementia may have followed at a later date. Thus, forgetfulness was not the first symptom they experienced.

Parkinson's type dementia was ruled out for my Mother. Recognizing the first symptom of a problem with an individual is often a great beginning point in the diagnosing process.

Early detection is very important. The earlier an individual is diagnosed with dementia of any sort, the better the life of that individual will be. The longer the individual goes without diagnosing and treating the disease, the more likely they will suffer more severe long-term consequences.

Many times the individual knows something is wrong. They are afraid to admit to the problem, which leads to a host of other problems. They may remove themselves from social situations for fear of embarrassment, and they can even become more susceptible to colds, flus, and viruses because they are not caring for themselves properly.

Another reason to support early diagnosis is the need to educate the caregivers. The more informed the caregivers are, the better they are equipped to care for their loved one. The better equipped they are, the happier both they and their loved one will be.

Lastly, the sooner medications are brought on board, the more effective they are. There are several medications used to treat Alzheimer's, and one size does not fit all. If one medication does not set well with an individual, another option needs to be investigated.

Momma began medication immediately after her diagnosis. She experienced zero side effects that I was aware of. I have only recently begun to realize that her medication is stealing her appetite. I CONSTANTLY question her as to what she has eaten every day. She wishes I would leave her alone, and I wish I didn't have to ask.

One of Momma's medicines is Aricept. After being on Aricept for about eighteen months, the doctor added Namenda to Momma's regiment. She remains on these two drugs today. However, it has been suggested that beginning these two drugs together is more effective in the long-run. The point to be made is this – seek medical help. Don't delay. Get it NOW!

HELP, we need a humor break!

Smile #4

My niece has recently been employed at a residential care facility. While preparing a resident for bed, my cute niece tucked the lady in and said, "Now you sleep good tonight." To which the lady responded, "I will if you get your Mac Truck big butt out of my room!" Except, she did NOT say "butt", if you get my point. My niece just laughed and kept on with her work.

Sometimes, you've just got to laugh!

# REVERSIBLE DEMENTIAS

Earlier I mentioned I prayed for my Momma to be diagnosed with a reversible dementia. I did not want her to have such a horrible disease. Just give us one of those reversible dementias, and we would get on with life. Unfortunately, dementia is not served a la carte, thus you are not given the option to pick and choose.

There are, however, reversible dementias. One of the most common reasons an individual might experience sudden onset symptoms of dementia is a side-effect of a medication.

A person does not wake up with Alzheimer's. You can wake up with the flu or a cold or a tummy ache, but you will not wake up with Alzheimer's. You might, however, wake up with dementia. This is referred to as "sudden onset dementia". In other words, you didn't have these symptoms yesterday. Remember, **dementia is the inability to think clearly which leads to difficulties with the activities of daily living.**

When this is the case, you must investigate the reason for the dementia. It is very likely you have a reversible dementia.

The first place to investigate as the source of this dementia is medication. Most all medications have side-effects that occur in one person or the other. As we age, the likelihood that a side-effect is dementia increases. One drug commonly known to cause hallucinations, and what I refer to as "strange talk", is Phenergan. This drug is often prescribed to calm an upset tummy, and it works wonderfully. However, it is not a drug of choice when physicians are prescribing for an elderly person. It will often give symptoms of dementia. Once the offending drug is removed, the symptoms of dementia leave, also.

Another reason an individual may have sudden onset symptoms of dementia is a vitamin B-12 deficiency. Once this deficiency is corrected, the dementia disappears. There is one small exception. If the vitamin B-12 deficiency has been in place for an extended period of time, the individual may not return to 100% capacity once the introduction of sufficient levels of vitamin B-12 appear. However, the improvement is substantial. I am currently caring for my mother-in-law, who has dementia because of an extremely low B-12 level. She is taking oral supplements and receiving shots. Her dementia is improving, but it is a very slow process.

If there is an infection in the body, sudden onset dementia can occur. This is one process God put in place to allow the body to scream "HELP!" One of the most common infections to cause dementia is a urinary tract infection. Once the infection has cleared, the dementia goes away.

One additional reason the individual might show sudden onset symptoms of dementia is the presence of a tumor somewhere in the body. Scriptures tell us we are "fearfully and wonderfully made" (Isaiah 139), and this is very true when you consider the body's response to a tumor. Once the tumor is removed, the symptoms of dementia leave.

The main point I want you to learn is this. When sudden onset symptoms of dementia appear, YOU MUST TAKE ACTION, IMMEDIATELY. This is the body's way of letting you know there is a situation that needs attention. Do not delay!

One last thought about the brain. The more you study and learn new pieces of information, the more synapses you build. The synapses become more tightly woven together. This is a great thing. One way to make a huge difference in the brain is to learn a foreign language. Since there is nothing about that language with which you are already familiar, everything you learn will be new. Your brain loves to be fed new information! Anyone interested in a little Pig Latin?

OK, now it is time to stand up, stretch the arms above your head, breathe deeply, and relax. You have been exercising your brain cells, and I am sure you are feeling a little tired. Take a short break, have a healthy snack, and let's keep learning together.

# IRREVERSIBLE DEMENTIAS

Now we are going to talk about the dementias that do not go away. While there are many diseases that cause irreversible dementias, Alzheimer's is the most common.

By the time we reach age 65, 10% of us will have Alzheimer's. By the time we reach age 85, 50% of us will have Alzheimer's. Those numbers are staggering and startling. I am a resident of South Carolina. In the year 2011, it was estimated that South Carolina had over 80,000 residents diagnosed with dementia.

As of this writing, there are an estimated 5.1 million Americans diagnosed with Alzheimer's, and there are over 15 million Americans providing care for someone with Alzheimer's. By the year 2050, those numbers are estimated to increase to 15 million Americans diagnosed and 45 million Americans providing care. If you do not presently know someone with Alzheimer's, let me assure you. You will soon! The numbers are not in your favor.

Let's not forget one important fact. The numbers just quoted only relate to Alzheimer's. There are other diagnoses that result in irreversible dementia. Huntington's Disease is a genetic defect on chromosome 4 in which nerve cells in certain parts of the brain waste away. Dementia is a symptom of Huntington's.

Pick's Disease can also show dementia as a

symptom. Pick's Disease is similar to Alzheimer's in that it affects memory and it is an irreversible disease. However, the first symptom of Pick's disease is NOT memory loss. Because the tissues in the temporal (the area around your ears) and frontal (forehead) lobes of the brain start to shrink, the most common symptom is often changes in behavior, speech difficulty, and impaired thinking. The frontal lobe is responsible for our ability to make socially acceptable decisions. When the frontal lobe is intact, we know what is appropriate and what is inappropriate. When the frontal lobe is diseased, the individual may have erratic behavior that is often socially unacceptable. These early personality changes can help doctors distinguish Pick's Disease from Alzheimer's.

Lewy Body Disease, AIDS, Parkinson's, and many other diseases can cause irreversible dementia. It is important to diagnose the individual properly. Assuming dementia is always a result of Alzheimer's is dangerous. For example, using Alzheimer's medication for an individual with Lewy Body Disease can prove to be detrimental to the individual. Once again, SEE YOUR DOCTOR!

There are many people who have dementia brought on by over 90 different diagnoses. It is imperative we learn all we can about dementia. This knowledge will make us better caregivers, bring a better quality of life to our loved one, and make our lives as caregivers more pleasant. It is a win-win situation! The motto for my company, Senior Life Journeys(www.seniorlifejourneys.com), is "Knowledge brings POWER. Power brings

HOPE, and hope brings SMILES. If there is one thing we all need, it is SMILES."

Smile #5

While caring for an elderly resident, the young woman asked the gentleman if he would like his long hair braided. He was very pleased at her offer, and he sat down for the service. Upon finishing, the young woman asked , "Will you please scoot up a bit so I can move out from behind you". Upon the request, the man moved his chair up quite a large amount. She commented, "Goodness, my rear end isn't THAT big!" "I know", he replied, "I've been looking at it!"

Sometimes, you've just got to laugh!

# WHAT ARE THE WARNING SIGNS?

According to the Alzheimer's Association (www.alz.org), which I hold as the most regarded professionals in the field, there are ten warnings signs of Alzheimer's. The list below is taken from their website, and I have "tweaked" it a little for my own purposes.

1.   Forgetfulness – This type of forgetfulness is often confused with common aging forgetfulness. With common aging, the individual will usually recall the information at a later time. However, with Alzheimer's, the individual will have little or no recollection of the information that was forgotten.

2.   Problems With Numbers – It is common for individuals to make mistakes in a checkbook or forget to pay a bill on time. The issue becomes more concerning when the problems occur frequently. The individual may also have difficulty staying on task long enough to get a job completed.

3.   Problems With Everyday Activities – It is common for an individual to find herself in a situation where she has forgotten how to do something she has done before. However, with Alzheimer's, this becomes a routine occurrence. Individuals may have problems driving to a familiar

location, operating a kitchen appliance, or remembering in which drawer certain clothing items are stored.

4. Problems Tracking Time and Place – If an individual awakens and does not know what day of the week it is, the knowledge will usually soon become evident. With Alzheimer's, this information remains an unknown. It is a reoccurring event. It is common for people with Alzheimer's to not recognize where they are or remember how they got there.

5. Problems With Vision – All of us experience changes in our vision as we age. Alzheimer's advances these changes. This may result in difficulty reading or even recognizing themselves in the mirror.

6. Lost Words – Stopping mid-sentence to search for a word, and not being able to retrieve that word, are symptoms of Alzheimer's dementia. It is not uncommon to forget a word. It is uncommon and concerning when this occurs frequently.

7. Lost Items – It is common for individuals with Alzheimer's to place personal belongings in an uncommon location. This makes it difficult for them, or their caregivers, to find the items. Of course, searching for the car keys is a common experience.

8. Poor Judgment – This is often demonstrated through the handling of money. For example, it is common to see large amounts of cash spent on television infomercials, donations to charities, or gifts to strangers. Everyone makes bad decisions, but Alzheimer's causes these bad decisions to appear more frequently.

9. Withdrawal – When a loved one does not want to participate in activities they would normally enjoy, this is a concerning symptom of Alzheimer's. This could also manifest itself in a lack of desire to participate in a hobby that was always enjoyable in the past.

10. Mood Changes – The mood of someone with Alzheimer's can change rapidly. They can also become irritated and confused very quickly. While it is not uncommon for a person to have a bad day, Alzheimer's intensifies those experiences.

**If your loved one is displaying signs of Alzheimer's, contact your doctor.**

When I recall the early days of Momma's diagnosis, I can see she displayed three of these ten warning signs. As I mentioned earlier, Momma was forgetful. We have already learned this is the hallmark symptom of Alzheimer's Dementia. Forgetfulness was, and still is, Momma's biggest issue.

Momma also had problems with numbers. The story of the bounced checks is evidence of that problem.

Lastly, Momma stopped sewing. My mother is a professional seamstress. She made every stitch of clothing my sisters and I wore, she wore, and even some of the clothes my daddy wore. At one point, she made a necktie for every man in our church for Christmas. Momma made draperies, placemats, and even upholstered furniture.

While working on a project one day, Momma had a difficult time threading the sewing machine. She asked me to take over the job. She blamed it on her vision. Which, by the way, is warning sign number five. I didn't think much of the situation, so I threaded the machine. The project continued as I expected.

When the next sewing project came up, Momma had a difficult time deciding how to turn the fabric to achieve a certain look. I knew then life had changed. Since that day, I have been in charge of the sewing machine. Momma is excellent at ironing seams, measuring, and encouraging me. However, her hands-on days are long gone. It is difficult for me to come to grips with this. There are projects I need her help to complete, and I am forced to figure them out without her input. It has caused me to learn, but it has caused me to be more aware of Momma's limitations. It does not make me sad for ME, but it makes me sad for HER. She wants to be able to sit down at the sewing machine and produce any object that might come to mind. She just is no longer able to do so.

Make sure you are aware of any changes that might be occurring in your loved one's life. It could be your observance that gets them the diagnosis they need to begin the treatment and medication that will be very helpful for their life.

Lastly, take the time to discern where your loved one fits on the ten warning signs list. How many of them apply? Can they dress themselves? Feed themselves? Ambulate? Toilet without help? Maintain personal hygiene? All of these answers will help your healthcare professional determine in what stage of the disease your loved one is living.

Smile #6

One of my favorite people at the assisted living where my mother lives use to say, "My remember-er doesn't work good at all. But my forgetter-er works GREAT." She learned it felt good to laugh. She even laughed at herself! Why?

Because...

Sometimes you've just got to laugh!

# WHAT ARE THE STAGES OF DEMENTIA?

It is important to understand the six stages of dementia. While Alzheimer's acts the same in the brain for everyone with the disease, dementia is as individualized as the person   There are stages of dementia that help us tract where in the disease process our loved one is living.

**Stage One** – Everything seems fine, but processing of information may be a little slower. The individual may feel blue, but they are still flexible and able to learn.   They like to have choices.  They can seem sharp and put together, but deep down there is a storm brewing.  Many times the individual knows something is "just not right", but they are not sure what is happening.  This is the most optimum time to see the doctor; however this seldom is the case.

**Stage Two** – This is the stage when we see individuals start to repeat themselves.  They seem to become less willing to adjust.  This may be due to their recognition of the problems they are experiencing.  They may seem hard and stubborn. They still hold authority figures in high esteem, and they still want to shine!

**Stage Three** -   These folks are always on the go.  They must always be doing something.  Others can recognize definite changes in them. They go back in time frequently, pulling on the memories that are most prominent and available. Their language skills are becoming vague, and they don't recognize their own flaws. They are often defensive. This is the stage where we often see Sundowner's Syndrome. Sundowner's is characterized by an extreme change in personality, often accompanied by hallucinations, when the sun goes down.

**Stage Four** – These people live in the moment and have a strong need for sensory stimulation. The lips, tongue, mouth, fingertips, palms, soles of feet, and genitalia are high sensory areas. They get caught in a moment of time, and they have no safety awareness. They are very focused on the here and now. What do I want? Do I like this? Me, Me, Me.

**Stage Five** – During this stage, we begin to notice a loss of fine motor skills in the eyes, hands, feet, and mouth. Coordination in fingers is declining, and feet do not move in a coordinated motion. This produces a high risk of falling. Weight loss and infections are common in this stage. Problems with chewing and swallowing become evident. There is no distinct speech, but they still have rhythm. Remember to slow down to their pace. Enjoy the MOMENT rather than pondering the event.

**Stage Six** – This is a sad stage. These folks are in the last stage of the disease. They pull within themselves. All we see is the outside, but there is much more to them. Their body is ruled by their reflexes and by muscles that are "turned on" all the time. It is common to see arms curled inward, legs pulled toward the body, and head bent down. This is because the muscles are never allowed to relax. Be cautious of the decision to force food and liquid. Doing so can cause them to aspirate. Allow the body to leave peacefully. It is good to say, "It is OK if you need to go. I will understand." Let go of what was and appreciate what is.

Since we have finished this chapter on a solemn note, I offer you this thought. Even in the final stages of any disease, it helps to remember this scripture, "I praise you because I am fearfully and wonderfully made; your works are wonderful, I know that full well. (Psalm 139:14)

# SO, WHAT HAPPENS TO
# THE BRAIN?

This information can be quite disturbing, but it is important knowledge. So, hang in there.

As we discussed earlier, the hippocampus is the first part of the brain to be affected by Alzheimer's. The hippocampus is that portion located in the center of the brain that is responsible first for receiving new information. As Alzheimer's begins to work its way through the brain, it camps out on the hippocampus and begins to cause it to shrink.

Along with the shrinkage, a gap begins to form around the hippocampus. This makes it difficult for new information to leave the "temporary file box", known as the hippocampus, and make its way to a permanent file box somewhere else in the brain. Because the hippocampus has started to shrink, this new information is lost. During the early stages of the disease, new information may be retained on one occasion and lost on another. As the disease progresses, new information is most always lost. I say "most always" because there is a notable exception. If that new information is accompanied by a very strong emotion, the information may be retained. Let me elaborate.

For the previous fifteen plus years, I have had the privilege of being the mother to a beautiful miniature dachshund named Pretzel. This little fellow has been the light of our lives for my husband, our daughter, my Momma, and myself. He had two back surgeries very early in his life, and he lived out his days in a wheelchair made especially for his cute little self. On March 10, 2011, Pretzel died. It was the most horrific experience of my life. I have experienced death in a loved one, but somehow this was different and has affected me in ways I cannot explain. It affected my entire family, and that would include Momma.

I had the unhappy task of telling Momma of Pretzel's death. She was very upset, and I so wanted to comfort her. We cried together, and we reminisced together. Momma has NOT forgotten this new information. A few days after his death, I planned a trip to Florida to grieve with our daughter. I told my mother repeatedly what time my flight left and what day I was returning. She could not retain this information. However, because the news of Pretzel's death was associated with deep grief and pain, she was able to retain the memory regarding his passing.

Knowing how information is processed in the brain of someone with Alzheimer's will help you understand your loved one better. Be patient with them. They have no control over the processes going on in their brain.

Think about that last statement a moment. Many people become very frustrated with their loved one when they have to repeat the same information many times or when the loved one tells the same story repeatedly. I wonder... if their loved one had heart disease, would they become angry when their heart did not work properly? If they had kidney failure, would they scream at their loved one because they could not urinate properly? Of course not. Yet, we often see caregivers yelling, "Momma, I have told you 49 times when your doctor's appointment is. Why don't you pay attention?"

It makes me cringe when I come across this situation. I am not a patient person. So, I want to pull them aside and give them a quick lesson in Alzheimer's and why their loved one is responding in this particular way. Alas, I can't enlighten the entire world. I am thrilled, however, that you are reading this book in an attempt to learn all you can. You are one of the enlightened people who will become a better caregiver in the future.

It's not quite time for a humor break, so let's keep going.

When Alzheimer's is present, the brain actually shrinks in size. By the time a person dies from the disease, the brain has most likely decreased to one-third of its original size. That would mean the individual has lost two-thirds of their brain matter. In addition, the brain matter that remains has holes, is not a healthy color, and is not functioning properly.

Alzheimer's is known for the plaque that develops on the brain. This plaque is different than the plaque on teeth or in arteries; however it might help to think about the damage it does in the brain as compared to the damage plaque does in an artery.

In an artery, the plaque keeps the blood from flowing properly. High cholesterol causes a build-up of this plaque, and the flow of blood is inhibited. Similarly, plaque on the brain causes damage with *the flow of information.*

Below is a picture that will help you see this more clearly. Instead of inserting here a drawing of neurons and branches from some highly renowned scientist, I have chosen the simplistic picture of gumballs that fell from a sweetgum tree to help you form a mental picture of plaque.

As you observe the picture, think of the gumballs as neurons in the brain. The healthy brain has over one hundred billion neurons. Each of these neurons has "little spikey things", much like the spikey things on the gumballs, and they are called

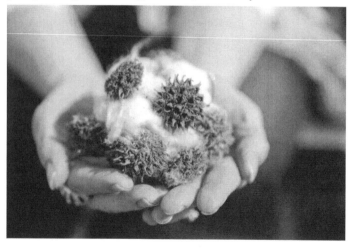

branches. We have over one hundred trillion of these branches. Information goes from one neuron to the other through a small electrical charge. When neurons connect to each other, it is referred to as a "synapse". When that connection is made, a release of chemicals occurs which are called neurotransmitters. The neurotransmitters carry the information to other neurons. Alzheimer's interrupts both this process of carrying information to other neurons (think gumballs) and the way neurotransmitters work.

Notice the white cotton balls between many of the gumballs. This represents the plaque known as beta-amyloid plaque. This plaque comes between the neurons and prevents the information from being moved around the brain. This plaque is composed of abnormal protein matter.

Scientists were successful in removing the plaque from Alzheimer's patients, however, once the plaque was removed, the disease continued to progress. Thus, it was not the cure they had hoped for.

Then there is TAU, which rhymes with cow. Tau is a substance that gets inside the neurons (think gumballs) and causes damage from the inside out. The inside of a neuron has nice straight paths. When tau invades, these paths become tangled, fall apart, and disintegrate. As a result, nutrients are not allowed to travel within the cells. This causes the death of the cell.

When you mix a shrinking hippocampus, holes in the brain, plaque around the neurons, and tau in the neurons, you have a good picture of Alzheimer's. There is so much more to learn. I HIGHLY recommend you visit the website of the Alzheimer's Association at www.alz.org . This is a site you can trust for reliable information. They also offer a toll-free hotline that is available 24/7. That number is 1-800-272-3900. I am proud to be an approved support group facilitator for the Alzheimer's Association South Carolina Chapter. When you visit their website, I recommend you find a support group near you.

Is your brain tired? You just used a large amount of the oxygen and fuel your blood carried to your brain while you were learning new information. In the day-to-day processes of life, your body sends 20 to 25 percent of the blood in your body to your brain. You use 20 percent of the oxygen and fuel that blood carries to go about your day. When you are learning new information, you may use up to 50 percent of the fuel and oxygen. So, there is a physiological reason for being tired.

The good news is the harder you think, and the more new information you learn, the more synapses are being formed in your brain. The more times you study that same information, the tighter those synapses become, and the more easily that information can be retrieved and reused. A good example of this would be practicing the piano. The first time you played a song, it was difficult, but a synapse was formed. The next time may have been a tiny bit easier. That is because another synapse was formed in the same area of the brain as the first synapse. As you continued to practice that piece of music, the synapses became stronger and more numerous. Finally, one day you could play the piece with no problem. When you have Alzheimer's, those synapses are not formed at all. So there is no way to retrieve the information that was learned the first time in order to build upon that knowledge.

Smile #7

While working with a senior citizen with dementia, the volunteer asked her if she would like to sing. The senior citizen motioned for the volunteer to get close enough to hear her whisper. "I don't want a man", she said. The volunteer was slightly shocked at the answer to her question regarding singing. "OK", she answered. The senior continued, "I don't think I can handle one. Do you?" Trying not to giggle, the volunteer politely agreed with the lady and recommended she sing instead. That seemed like a great option, and the senior was happy to join the fun.

It was a fun moment for the senior to sing, but it was a great moment for the volunteer to experience with the senior. A little laughter, a little light-heartedness, and a little smiling go a long way in making us better caregivers. It is OK to laugh at the funny things your loved ones says or does. So, lighten up a little and enjoy life.

Sometimes, you've just got to laugh!

# THE BRAIN HAT

I am a hands-on type learned, so I use props when I educate about dementia. It seems to help people learn more easily when they can hear **and** see the information being taught. That is the reason the brain hat came into existence; see the picture below. I created and use this little hat almost every time I speak to a group or coach on a one-on-one basis.

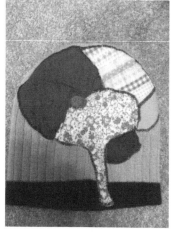

It is not likely your brain is divided into sections by such colorful fabrics, but wouldn't it be fun if it were? "Carol, I am diagnosing you with a problem in the blue flowered section." This hat represents a cross-section of the brain. The eye would be located to the left of the brown section on the left side of the hat. Instead of blue flowered, the doctor would refer to that section as the *medulla oblongata*. That is where we will start. An important and interesting fact leads me to start with the *medulla oblongata*. This is the part of the brain you cannot live without. Let's work our way through the brain in a counter clockwise direction. The further around the circle we travel, the degree of necessity for survival each part holds becomes evident. In other words, we cannot live without the blue flowered part, but we can live without the brown part. Let's see why.

As stated above, the flowered section on the brain hat is the medulla oblongata. I just love saying "medulla oblongata". Try it. It rolls off your tongue quite nicely and makes you sound so intelligent.

The medulla oblongata is responsible for things you don't have to think about in order to live. These functions are called autonomic functions. For instance, this is the part of the brain that controls respirations, digestion, and heart rate. It is also the relay station for nerve signals going to and from the brain.

The next section of the brain is the cerebellum. This section is blue on the brain hat. The cerebellum is responsible for movement, coordination, posture, and balance.

Travel on around the brain hat, and you will reach the green section. This is the occipital lobe of the brain. The visual cortex is located here, so it is responsible for vision and the processing of that vision.

The pink patterned section is the parietal lobe. It is responsible for our ability to control orientation of location. In other words, when you reach for an object, you know where to place your hand to grasp that object. You will not reach to the left or the right; you will place your hand squarely on the object. In addition, it helps us determine the speed in which an object might be moving. This is important in many parts of our lives, but it is especially important if you are a driver. It is also used to help in recognition of speech. Also, this section is responsible for our ability to process pain and touch from the skin and internal organs. So, if you have a tummy ache or a headache, your parietal lobe is relaying that information.

As we continue on around the brain in a counter clockwise pattern, we next come upon the frontal lobe. This is the part of the brain that was removed in past ages and called a lobotomy. You can live without the temporal lobe, but we might not want to be around you! This part of the brain is responsible for judgment and impulse control. It tells you it is inappropriate to run naked through the grocery store or tell dirty jokes at church. It is also involved in emotion, memory and speech.

The frontal lobe is the last portion of the brain to develop, and does not fully develop until we are young adults. That would explain why a teenager will do things that cause an adult to wonder why they acted in a certain way. "What were they thinking?" is the question we often ask. In actuality, their brain was not capable of processing that information in a logical manner, as the frontal lobe was not fully developed. The ability to reason and problem solve are not strong suits of a young person until the frontal lobe has matured. Lastly, our ability to feel the pain of others is processed in the frontal lobe.

As we continue this journey on the brain hat, we come back to the flowered part. The rounded portion of the flowered part is the temporal lobe. I should have made it a different color! However, the temporal lobe can easily be identified as that area that hurts when you get a headache in the "temple" region of the head – or just above the ears. It will not surprise you to know the auditory cortex is located in this region, so sound sensation is processed in the left-temporal lobe. Language recognition is also processed here.

Lastly, we come to the blue fuzzy ball in the middle of the hat. That is where we will concentrate our study. First, though, we seriously need a humor break. Remember how we learned your brain uses more oxygen and fuel when you are concentrating? If you are like me, most of this information was "news" to you, so you used a ton of oxygen and fuel. A humor break is in order.

Smile #8
A resident of a care facility was happy to announce she had found her missing dentures. She had safely stored them . . . in the tank of the TOILET!

Sometimes you've just got to laugh!

Now, back to the hippocampus, the blue fuzzy ball in the middle of the brain hat. When a person is diagnosed with Alzheimer's type dementia, the first symptom displayed is usually that of memory loss. This problem began in the hippocampus, or cardboard file box. New information enters the brain and first lands on the hippocampus. It is placed inside the cardboard file box in an appropriate file folder. In time, that information is moved from the file (the hippocampus) to a steel file drawer. This steel file drawer is represented by another portion of the brain. When Alzheimer's has entered the hippocampus, the information cannot be stored. The hippocampus has been undergoing serious malformation. It has begun to shrink, and a gap is forming around the lobe. The information may land on the hippocampus, but it cannot stay there. Since it cannot stay there, it cannot move to another portion of the brain (the steel file drawer). The information is lost forever.

When you tell your loved one the same information repeatedly, they are not forgetting it on purpose. They do not ask you, "Honey, where is the bathroom?" repeatedly, just to see if they can irritate you. They honestly have no idea where the bathroom is located. That information has not landed in the brain's files.

Remember the head of cauliflower? Recall, also, the knowledge that the brain, as a whole, shrinks to one-third its original size. The brain gets large holes throughout it. Lastly, the brain is attacked by beta-amyloid plaque and tau. When all these things come together, you have a clear picture of Alzheimer's.

The more you understand what is going on inside your loved one's brain, the better you will be at providing care. The better you are at giving the care needed, the higher quality of life you and they will have.

# THE HAM SANDWICH

Is there anyone on the planet who has never had a problem with communication? Lack of communication destroys marriages, causes business ventures to fail, and sends people to counselors and psychiatrists. We all need to communicate on some level in order to exist.

If you think communication is difficult in everyday life, add dementia to the situation. As dementia progresses, the areas of the brain that are responsible for communication are affected, also. The dementia causes the individual to begin experiencing a loss of words. The words that come naturally to all of us are scrambled and often lost completely when Alzheimer's enters the picture.

There are techniques to be learned that will aid us in communicating with our loved ones. Let's begin with a few simple, but extremely important, points of courtesy.

Do not EVER approach an individual from behind. In actuality, we should never do this with anyone. There are not too many people who enjoy being startled. Being startled is especially uncomfortable for someone with Alzheimer's. Why is it worse for them? Their peripheral vision has decreased dramatically. (We will discuss this in a later chapter.) While the average person may be aware of someone approaching from the side, the individual with Alzheimer's has no such awareness.

Be careful to approach them from the front.

While still ten feet away, extend your arm and hand in greeting, and begin speaking to the individual. Be aware of the response you receive from the individual you are approaching. If they do NOT extend their arm to grasp your hand, then respect their need for privacy and remain several feet away. If they extend their hand, you can assume they are welcoming you to enter their "private space" to the extent of the length of their arm. If they bend their arm, thus pulling you closer to them, it is appropriate to approach them in a more intimate way.

What is the best way to begin communication? I am so glad you asked. I grew up in the South, and I attended many church services. We all knew how to shake hands, and we were excellent at throwing a covered dish supper. Both of these come to mind when I am working with a friend with Alzheimer's.

When shaking hands, the hand positioning is different. I refer to the proper hand position as a "Ham Sandwich". That sticks in my brain because us Southerners love food. Find an unsuspecting friend in order to take this handshake on a trial run. Extend your right hand to their right hand, and place the webbing between your thumb and index finger into the same webbing on their hand. When the fingers relax, they are resting on the palm and wrist of the other person's hand.

Think of your hand as a piece of bread. Think of your friend's hand as the ham inside the sandwich. Now, place your other hand on the outside of your friend's hand. That completes the sandwich with a second piece of bread. Your hands are two pieces of bread, and their hand is the ham. Voila – a HAM SANDWICH!

Why go to this effort? For a few reasons. Believe it or not, it is possible to have the bones in your hand broken by a totally unsuspecting old lady who shakes your hand. She looks so innocent and frail, but when she reaches for your hand, the squeeze is on! All of a sudden, you have broken bones, and she has no idea she has caused you pain. When the ham sandwich handshake is employed, the chances of hurting someone are greatly reduced.

Along that same train of thought, it is easy for a caregiver to bruise the hand of an elderly person with a normal handshake. If you look at the skin on the back of a twenty-year old hand, it is taught. When you pull up on the skin, a small amount lifts, and it returns to the hand very tightly. If you lift in the same spot of a seventy year old hand, it is very loose, and it does not return to the hand in a taught way. As we age, the fat padding on the back of our hands goes away. This leaves skin and bone with no fat to protect us. Shaking hands in a normal fashion could easily result in a bruise on the back of the hand of an elderly person.

Another advantage to the ham sandwich handshake is in regards to pressure points in the palm of the hand. There are many pressure points in the hand that aid in relaxation. The positioning of the hands in the ham sandwich aid in placing pressure in the palm of the hand, and this helps both you and the individual relax.

Smile #9

One night while bathing my two year old daughter, she proudly announced, "Momma, I just washed my three head!" She was proud. I was confused. "You washed your three head? Do it again so I can see!" Of course, she washed her forehead. Three head or "four head", it was just funny!

Sometimes, you've just got to laugh.

# EYE TO EYE CONTACT

Now that you have mastered the ham sandwich handshake, let's take it to the next level. I want to preface this section with a warning. The technique you are about to learn will aid you in working with everyone you know, and if someone uses these techniques on YOU, be aware, they are powerful techniques in effective communication.

I employed these techniques while approaching my husband over the need to replace the refrigerator. I will tell you about that later.

Once you have extended your hand at a ten foot distance, been invited closer into the private space of an individual, and employed the ham sandwich handshake, you are now in a position for intimate conversation. At this point, you are most likely standing, and your loved one is probably sitting. This is NOT the most effective way to begin communication. Before you get close enough to touch them, you have already announced yourself and greeted them. You want to make the time you will spend communicating as effective as possible.

Start by kneeling beside your loved one on their dominant side. If they are left-handed, kneel on their left side. Likewise, if they are right-handed, kneel on their right side. If you are positioned on their dominant side, the brain will respond more favorably to the information you are about to give them. This is an easy change in our approach, but a very effective change, indeed.

Why do we kneel? If you are in a seated position, and someone enters your private space and remains in a standing position while talking to you, you have to look up to have eye-to-eye contact. This position is physically uncomfortable. It also places the standing person in an assumed position of authority. "I am above you. You have to look UP to me." When you desire meaningful and effective conversation with anyone, this type of posture is not recommended. So, simply kneel on the dominant side of the person you are wishing to speak with.

Now that you are in place to begin conversation, you can shift the position of your left hand. Here are a few ideas. Use your left hand to rub the back of their hand. It is not uncommon to see the loved one sit with their shoulders lifted towards their ears. They are often tense, and cold.

Individuals with Alzheimer's burn calories at a rapid rate. While the average individual sleeps, they burn approximately 200 calories. The individual with Alzheimer's burns 600 calories sleeping. Compare that with the number of calories you burn walking down the hall and the number of calories your loved one with Alzheimer's burns walking down the hall. This high fuel burning rate causes the individual to be cold.

In addition to burning calories, the loss of an insulating fat pad in many places of the body causes the individual to be colder than normal. Therefore, this rubbing of the back of their hand will warm them a bit. If you are observant, you will often see their shoulders lower and their respirations slow a bit. When this occurs, their ability to concentrate on your words is increased.

Another idea is to place your left hand on their shoulder or leg. If you feel close enough to the individual, rub that shoulder or leg. If that is too intimate, rubbing the hand is most always appropriate. Please give consideration to your relationship with the individual in regards to how you touch them.

Now, let me tell you how all this can be used to your benefit in everyday life with a real life example. My refrigerator was dying a slow and painful death. The frozen fruits were no longer frozen, and the water in the refrigerator was no longer cold. My husband kept saying I had left the door open or I had too many items in the freezer to allow the air to move around the food. Blah, Blah, Blah! That was what I thought. After a few days, I placed myself on his left side (he is a lefty), took his hand, rubbed it gently, and said,

"Michael, the refrigerator is dying. Unless you want your chicken to turn green, we probably should purchase a new one."

I continued to look him in the eyes and rub his hand. He gently replied,

"Babe, I think you should go buy the refrigerator you want."

I responded, "But the one I want is not inexpensive."

To which he replied, "I know. Just make sure you get exactly what you want."

This technique works like a charm. Every time I open my new refrigerator, I think about dementia.

I have decided to call my beautiful appliance my "dementia refrigerator". Remember, however, when someone is using these techniques on YOU, it is imperative you be aware of their power!

# PLEASE, DON'T TELL ME
# THAT STORY **AGAIN**!

"Did I tell you I am from North Carolina?"

"No," her friend responded.

"Well, I am.  I went back there last week.  I drove and drove, and I could not find the house I grew up in.  I know you are suppose to go by Gibson's Grocery Store, turn right across the railroad tracks, and the house should be just around the corner.  But, it was not there. "

A few minutes later, the lady returned and said to her friend, "Did I tell you I am from North Carolina?"

"No" her friend responded.

"Well, I am.  I went back there last week.  I drove and drove, and I could not find the house I grew up in.  I know you are suppose to go by Gibson's Grocery Store, turn right across the railroad tracks, and the house should be just around the corner.  But, it was not there. "

Slightly frustrated at hearing the story yet again, the friend removed herself from sight of the lady.  It did not work.  Finding the friend down the hall, the lady said, "Did I tell you I am from North Carolina?"

This time the friend responded, "Yes, you did."

"I did NOT tell you.  Who told you?  I bet it was that damn woman across the hall.  She just can't keep her mouth shut.  I swear these people really get on my nerves."

The friend was shocked at the language the lady used, and she was disturbed at how visibly distraught the woman became.

This scene is played out day after day by people with dementia. They will tell the same story again, and again, and again, and again....well, you get the idea. What is the best way to handle this?

Instead of responding with "yes, you did" when asked for the third time if she had mentioned she was from North Carolina, a better response would have been, "tell me about it". Those are magical words. They work in many situations. Why are they magical? They say neither "yes" or "no" to a question, and they allow the story teller the dignity of telling their story AGAIN.

As dementia progresses, the mind goes back in time. The date and time in which you are living is NOT the date and time in which the person with dementia is living. They will not and cannot enter your world. You must enter their world. Let me say that again, with emphasis. **They will not and cannot enter your world. You must enter their world.** If you become frustrated, the individual will be frustrated. If you are patient, listen to the story for the forty-seventh time, they will be happy to tell it for what they are sure is the first time.

Another good reason to listen to their story repeatedly is a sad one. As the dementia progresses, they will not be able to repeat their stories. You will wish you could hear the story about grandpa and the cow, or Momma and the peanut butter, or whatever the story may be, and they will no longer be able to tell you. So, let them tell the stories while they are able. Listen. Smile. Be patient. It is NOT about you. IT IS ALL ABOUT THEM!

# WHAT IF THEY ASK THE SAME QUESTION REPEATEDLY?

I giggled under my breath when I wrote that title. Why? Because I can guarantee your loved one WILL ask the same question repeatedly. I can also guarantee it will get on your nerves if you don't understand what is going on inside their brain or you don't have a plan on how best to respond.

Let's review. The hippocampus is the part of the brain responsible for obtaining and processing new information. Alzheimer's has been doing its dirty work on the hippocampus of the individual diagnosed, and they CANNOT retain new information. No matter how hard they try, that new information will not take root anywhere in the brain. That would explain the following conversation.

"Momma, you have a doctor's appointment at 2:00 today."

"I do? I didn't know that."

"Yes, I will take you to the doctor for a 2:00 appointment."

About five minutes later …

"Are we doing anything important today," Momma asks.

"Yes, you have a doctor's appointment at 2:00 today."

"I do? Well, why haven't you told me about this earlier? I could have had my hair done."

"I just told you not more than five minutes ago. You forgot. You forget everything."

"You did not tell me! If you had, I would have remembered! I AM NOT CRAZY! If you would treat me right, we would not have these problems."

And then the frustrations mount on both sides, the anger increases on both sides, and the tension becomes palpable. Let's discover a way to prevent that frustration from building.

The part of the brain engaged in listening is the auditory cortex, and it is located in the temporal lobe. The part of the brain involved in seeing is located in the occipital lobe in the back of the brain. When we combine both verbal communication and physical cues by using a little bit of charades, we actually engage two parts of the brain rather than just one. This doubles our chances of reaching our loved one with the information we need to present.

Let's look at the same conversation in a different light.

We might say, "Momma, we are going to the doctor at two o'clock today." Momma might remember this information for a few minutes. We have given her the verbal information, only, and we have activated the auditory cortex of the brain. If instead of merely telling Momma this information we did a little gesturing, it might look like this.

Positioned in front of Momma, eye to eye contact, hand over hand, we say, "Momma, you have a doctor's appointment at two o'clock today." We then place two fingers in the air. This will give her a visual cue as to what two o'clock means. When we speak of going somewhere, we could act out driving a car. Relaying the information in both verbal and visual forms is useful in helping the brain retain the information. Think "charades" when relaying information.

These same visual cues can be used to the detriment of a situation, also. Let's pretend the following situation has occurred. You have arrived to visit Dad, and you find him sitting alone in his room. You might say, "Daddy, did you have lunch today?" Daddy may or may not answer the question. If, however, you are shaking your head "yes" while asking the question, Daddy is probably going to pick up on the visual cue of your head moving in the "yes" motion and respond with "yes". This may or may not be the correct answer. However, Daddy is merely responding to his environment.

"Daddy, did they remember to take you down to Bingo today," she says while shaking her head "no" the entire time. "I bet you didn't get to play Bingo, did you?" Still shaking her head "no", Daddy responds with "No" as a definitive answer. In fact, Daddy played Bingo and won $75, a pair of socks, and a bag of chips!

Smile #10

While caring for an elderly woman deep in the throes of dementia, the caregiver was pleased to welcome the woman's husband for regular "huggy time" visits. They would hug and kiss and giggle. Upon his leaving each and every time, the lady would ask, "Who is that man?" The caregiver would reply, "He is your husband." To which the elderly woman would say, "I have a husband? Well, he sure is ugly!"

Sometimes you've just got to laugh!

# I TALK LIKE A TRUE SOUTHERNER, AND THAT AIN'T SO GOOD

I like the word "ain't". It has a way of making a point that no other word is quite capable of doing.

I hail from The Great State of South Carolina. Though I was born in Florida, I grew up in North Carolina and am a southerner through and through. I talk like a southerner, also. I am sure you have picked up on some of my southern phrases through the reading of this book. I hope you are inspired to adopt some of them for your own edification!

Many people think southerners talk with a drawl. They assume we all sound like Scarlett O'Hara. Well, we don't. A good southerner can rattle off twice as many words per minute as anybody else on the planet. When we are excited, we can "let it rip", as us South Carolinians might say. If you are not from around our neck of the woods (I will let you figure out what that means), then you just need to listen quicker. Once you master that skill, you will be able to keep up with our conversations.

This is all well and good and perfectly acceptable. Except...when you are talking to someone with dementia. If you are talking quickly, you are going to diminish their ability to comprehend and understand what you are saying. Remember, the brain is diseased. It cannot perform the same tasks the healthy brain is capable of. Words become scrambled. If you are speaking quickly, this just complicates matters for them. Take the time to look the individual in the eye while calmly and slowly relaying your information.

Many times the individual will search for the proper word, and a totally new word will escape from their lips. This makes conversation extremely difficult. Let's look at an example of a scrambled word conversation.

"Hey, John. I need a tromby."

"Hi, Dad. Did you say you need a tromby."

"Yes, get me a tromby."

John replies, "Help me remember, Dad. What do you do with a tromby?"

Dad seemed a little confused, but he answered with, "You know. You use a tromby to make your hair look good."

"Oh yeah. I remember."

Of course, Dad was looking for a comb. However, the word was lost from his vocabulary, and the only word he could think of was tromby. John could have responded with, "Dad, I don't know what a tromby is. For heaven's sake. Why don't you learn to talk correctly?" This would have made for a very unpleasant moment and a difficult situation. In addition, Dad's needs would not have been met.

Fortunately, John had excellent dementia communication skills. Rather than attacking his dad, he accepted responsibility for not knowing what his dad needed. He said, ""Help me remember, Dad. What do you do with a tromby?" This may have caused John to feel silly, but it didn't cause Dad any embarrassment; it made for a more manageable situation for both John and Dad. John also repeated his dad's request. Dad was comforted to know John was listening.

It is also important to watch the physical clues Dad might be offering. While explaining to John of his need for a tromby, Dad may have been running his fingers through his hair. This is a great clue for John.

Sometimes the situation requires a little more in-depth delving for information. The question may need to be asked, "What do you do with a tromby?" "What color is your tromby?" Ask questions as if you are totally aware of what a tromby is and own one yourself. After all, you probably do. YOU just didn't know it was called a tromby.

If the conversation is totally scrambled, it might sound like this.

"I need the one with the one and the other that you know for yesterday."

"Mom, you need the one with the one?" Is that right?

"Well, yes. You should know that. Why can't you understand what I am trying to say....I need the ONE! Get it!"

Many times this will require the caregiver to provide a distraction in a major way. What we want to avoid is a confrontation on any level. It is best to have supportive communication. Being confrontational will NEVER prove beneficial. We will discuss more about how to distract someone in a later section. However, Mom could be helped through this particular situation by changing the subject to one that is happy and acceptable to both parties.

Smile #11

Mr. William Root raised and sold pigs. However, pig sales were slow, and he pondered this issue. He felt he needed to advertise, but he was stunned at the effectiveness of his sign. It read, "PIGS FOR SALE" – Will Root.

Sometimes, you've just got to laugh!

# FOUR LETTER WORDS, AND I'M NOT TALKING ABOUT L-O-V-E

When your loved one becomes agitated or feels confronted, there is a good chance you will hear words that make you uncomfortable. This is especially true if that loved one spent their life avoiding those words. It can be a very disturbing event if you do not understand what is happening in their brain.

Remember the brain hat from our earlier study? The brown part of the brain is the frontal lobe. This is where inhibitions are stored. The frontal lobe helps us know what is appropriate and what is inappropriate. Saying certain words in certain situations is definitely inappropriate. When dementia becomes part of the picture, the ability to discern appropriate and inappropriate is often lost. This is why an individual might use those four letter words.

Another reason is the location of those four letter words in the brain. The information we learned early in our life is stored in a different part of our brain than the information we learned recently. Most all of us learned these taboo words somewhere between age two and seven. This is the same time we learned words regarding sex and racial slurs. Most likely, we were admonished the first few times we used these words, or maybe we had our mouths washed out with soap. This caused us to push the words to "the back of our brain". They were not words we used every day. By the time we reached age seven to ten, we learned the art of word substitution. Therefore, the words were not used frequently.

Dementia takes away common words, and they are the words first lost. Remember the story of Jim's Dad calling a comb a tromby? He had lost the word "comb". However, it is very likely Jim's Dad could have easily recalled many four letter words that might have shocked those listening. Those words were not everyday words for him, and they were stored in a different part of his brain. Therefore, he could recall them.

This explains why good people begin cursing. I have a friend whose mother's favorite word is "hell". She "hells" everything from the situation, to the bread, to the chair, to the weather. "Hell, I don't want to eat dinner." It makes my friend cringe, but she realizes it is the disease talking – not her mother.

My grandmother, Bessie, was a dedicated Christian woman. She raised three boys and three girls, and she did so without the use of inappropriate words. If her children ever considered using those words, they certainly were punished. As Grandma's Alzheimer's progressed, she stopped speaking. My Aunt Evelyn began to pray, "Lord, please just let Mother speak again. I want to hear her voice." Well, God has a big sense of humor. He honored my aunt's heartfelt request, and my grandmother spoke. She was seated at the dinner table, and suddenly Grandma said, "Evelyn! I haven't pooped in a year." Except Grandma didn't say "pooped", if you catch my drift. Well, Aunt Evelyn just about fell on the floor laughing her head off, and saying words of thanksgiving – all at the same time. See, I told you God has a sense of humor!

It is also not unusual to hear statements like, "Are you pregnant? You sure look pregnant." Or, "Do something about your hair. It looks awful." These statements are not intended to be hurtful. People with mid to advanced stage dementia often say what comes to mind with no thought whatsoever as to how those words come across.

It just doesn't matter. That is a fact. IT JUST DOESN'T MATTER. Do not correct or admonish them for cursing. It is not them talking. It is the disease talking. If you correct them, you have just put yourself in a position of authority over them, and that is not a position they are willing to give you or one to which they will submit.

Let it go. Relax. Laugh, if appropriate. It will be OK. Even if those words come out in a setting that is formal, just smile, nod, and act like nothing happened.

Now, If your loved one spent their life using those four letter words as a matter of routine, and dementia becomes part of their future, they will likely no longer curse.

I find this amusing. I have spent my life trying hard to avoid using swear words. They are not a part of my everyday vocabulary. Therefore, if I get dementia, I might be heard swearing frequently. My sister, on the other hand (I love you, Sissy!), has not been as cautious in her choice of words. I am guessing we might end up sitting next to each other in our elder years with me cussing like crazy, and my sister sitting quietly. Because most people do not understand what happens in the human brain, they will assume I just have a potty mouth! Geez! It just isn't fair.

Smile #12

Daddy wanted to teach his young son a few life-skills, thus the day was spent in the field learning how to construct a sturdy fence. Dad said, "You see this nail? Grab the hammer. When I nod my head, you hit it." The young boy did exactly as instructed. Guess Daddy needed to be careful how he worded instructions!

Sometimes, you've just got to laugh!

# MORE TIPS FOR COMMUNICATING

Communicating with our loved ones with dementia is so important. We must employ every technique available, and be on the lookout for techniques that work best with OUR loved one.

A great technique to employ is to repeat the question back to your loved.

Mom might say, "Are we going to have lunch?"

You know you just finished lunch, but Mom doesn't seem to remember this. The common response would be, "Mom, we just ate lunch. Don't you remember?" Let me pause a moment and ease your mind. You WILL use the words, "Don't you remember?" more times than you can believe. They will escape from your lips before you can retrieve them. Then you think, "How crazy am I? Of course she doesn't remember! She has dementia." I know, because I have done this too many times to count. Ease up on yourself. This type of statement is one we use routinely in our lives. It is a habit, but it is one that you can work to change.

A better response might be, "Are you asking when we will eat again?" You have rephrased her question, and repeated it back to her. This will allow you to say, "Mom, we will eat at 5PM. There are about four more hours before we have supper. Do you think you would like a cracker or some popcorn to help with the hunger?"

Now Mom is satisfied that you heard her, you responded to her, and she can have a snack. It calms the situation, and no one had to become agitated or irritated. Redirecting and refocusing are keys to good communication.

This makes me think of the technique my mother always used with my two sisters and me when we were growing up. We would ask Momma a question, and she would answer with, "You can ask your Daddy when he gets home." I can guarantee you she was totally aware we would NEVER ask our Daddy when he got home. That answer always frustrated me, and I managed to muster the courage to argue back. "I want to know what YOU think the answer is. I don't want to wait until Daddy gets home." Of course, Momma never gave in, and that technique usually meant I had to drop the subject.

In actuality, this is part of Diversion Therapy. It is not saying "no", and it is not saying "yes". One of my husband's favorite answers to a question is, "Yes, maybe later." Of course, who knows when "later" will ever arrive, but he has ended the conversation on a positive note.

"Carol, are you going to take me to get my nails manicured? "

"Yes, Momma. Maybe later."

This will usually suffice as an answer, and it is simple and easy to navigate. While thinking about ending a conversation on a positive note, let's look at the opposite.

Ending a conversation on a negative note is never fun. This type situation should be avoided in all of life, especially when living with dementia. This negativity can come from the person with dementia or from the caregiver.

"You look fat! Are you pregnant?" Of course, these words are hurtful. However, the person saying those words did not intend to be hurtful at all. These words are coming from a diseased brain. That disease has drastically affected the frontal lobe of the brain, and that person has no control over what is appropriate and what is acceptable. These words are not coming from the person you know and love. It is the disease talking – not the person. This can be hard to accept when the hurtful words are being said to you.

We might respond back with, "That is a really mean thing to say. Why would you be so nasty to me?" This is a useless response. It is very likely the person will now become defensive, and the comment that should have been ignored has now turned into a battle.

A better response might be, "I might need to eat more celery instead of doughnuts. Do you like peanut butter on your celery?" Here we have used diversion therapy to change the subject and to avoid confrontation.

Always try to leave your conversation on a positive note. One of the questions I am known for asking is, "How did you leave the situation?" It is important that we leave the situation on a positive note.

Remember, the brain with dementia is more likely to remember information that has a strong emotion attached to it. If you have angered or frustrated them, this emotion might cause the information to stick around. The opposite is true, also. If you bring them information that is attached to a happy or excited emotion, they are more likely to remember the information. That being said, let's do our best to leave our loved one with a happy or excited memory.

Smile #13

Husbands are interesting. Take for instance the man who called his wife and asked for her phone number.

Sometimes, you've just got to laugh!

# DON'T PUSH BACK

If you were to place your hand against a brick wall and push with all your might, that brick wall would remain steady and unmovable. I want you to have that image in your mind the next time you even *think* about arguing with your loved one with dementia. Just as surely as the brick wall is not moving, no matter how determined and persistent you may be, your loved one is not going to change his mind. He knows what he knows, and you are just plain WRONG.

Confabulation is defined by Wikipedia as: "a memory disturbance that is characterized by verbal statements and/or actions that inaccurately describe history, background, and present situations". That is a great definition. The individual with dementia, especially in the latter stages, will tell stories that have little to no truth in them. Many times the listener is unaware the story is false, but often times the listener realizes the story is wrought with inaccuracies. It is at this point we have a tendency to correct the individual. Don't Do It!

The storyteller is not intentionally telling a lie. They are totally unaware the story is inaccurate. They are telling the story as truthfully as they are capable of doing. In their mind, the facts are being relayed exactly as they happened. However, the story has been manufactured in their brain, and telling them they are wrong is a complete waste of time. Not only is it a waste of time, it will frustrate you and make them angry or even sad. It is a good way to agitate them.

What should you do? Listen. That is such an easy thing to do. You can shake your head in agreement, use words like "really, WOW, and tell me more" without ever hinting you may not believe the story. The storyteller gets to talk, you listen, and all is well in the world.

Let me give you a great example of this "confabulation" in action. I had a friend in the very late stages of dementia who always introduced herself as the wife of the chief of police of a nearby town. I had no reason not to believe her, so I took this story to be a fact. It never occurred to me it could be inaccurate. One day I mentioned to some friends that this lady's husband was the chief of police, and a gentleman responded, "No he wasn't. She was NEVER married!" I was shocked.

While visiting with this same lady some time later, I discovered she was now "married" to a man who lived in the same facility. The next day, she was "married" to a different man. It was always interesting to see how many men she had "married", but they all made her happy.

Isn't that the point? Her stories and her "marriages" all made her happy. I was glad to go along with her; she was glad to tell her stories, and we both left the situation with a smile. Of course, this same lady told me she loved me so much she was going to "slap my dimples off my face". Hmmm, glad she didn't try that!

The point remains; "pushing back" is never

beneficial. Going with the flow, moving as they move, or "dancing" with them in a verbal way is always your best plan. Be cooperative. In fact, that is good advice for all life. Do you know anyone who enjoys being corrected? It is often beneficial to just go with the flow, rather than pushing back, even when the individual has no cognitive deficits.

Remember, just because you are correct, doesn't mean the outcome is going to be good. Having a good outcome is what is important.

# DIVERSION THERAPY

This may sound a bit foreign to you, but if you have or have ever cared for children, you have practiced diversion therapy. It looks something like this.

"I WANT THAT TRUCK!" Little Johnny screams.

"Johnny, that is Peter's truck. You need to let him play with it for a while."

"BUT IT WANT IT, NOW! WHA! WHA! WHA!"

"Johnny, I know you want the truck, but let me show you the really neat red car that I just bought yesterday."

This, of course, worked wonderfully, and Little Johnny's attention was diverted from the truck to the red car.

My friend, Sarah, was a lovely woman whom I enjoyed visiting. Sarah, however, was in the late stages of dementia, and she left this world much too soon for my liking. Each time I visited Sarah, our conversation would always turn towards the same train of thought. Sarah wanted to go home.

It was Sarah's belief her mother was waiting on her because she had supper ready and waiting. We will learn in a later chapter how the brain actually begins to exist in a different date and time, and that is exactly what had happened to Sarah. As best I could tell, Sarah thought she was about 10-15 years old, and her mother was going to be upset if Sarah did not arrive home soon. Therefore, she would always ask, "Will you please take me home? Momma has dinner ready, and she is going to be mad if I don't get there soon."

At this point in our conversation, I could have easily replied, "Sarah, honey, your Momma died in 1957. She is not waiting on you to arrive home and eat supper."

While this statement would have been true, it would not have been kind. As we will learn in the chapter on "Therapeutic Fibbing", sometimes we might need to alter the facts a little to navigate a particular situation. So a better response to Sarah was, "Sarah, I'm really hungry, also. What do you think your Momma cooked for dinner? Do you think she has pot roast and potatoes? "Of course, Sarah most likely had a response of some sort. I then moved Sarah further and further away from the thought of going home to Momma.

"Well," Sarah might say, "Momma makes a good pot roast."

"Does she fix mashed potatoes and gravy with that pot roast?"

"Yes she does."

"I want to tell you what I had for supper last night, Sarah. I had scrambled eggs and toast for SUPPER. Don't you think that is a strange thing to have for supper?"

"If that is what you want, I don't care what you eat", Sarah might respond with her typical sharp humor.

"Have you ever eaten eggs and toast for

supper? I once even ate frog legs. Can you believe that?"

The conversation is now about food, and it steers further and further away from "Momma". Sarah is not upset, she is not being ignored, and her intellect is being challenged to the degree in which she is capable of participating. It is a win-win situation all the way around!

Asking to go home is a common theme for conversations when you visit someone in the late stages of dementia. It is a "hot topic", and should always be handled gingerly.

"You look like a nice lady. Will you please take me home? I want out of this place!"

"I am absolutely willing to help you. You can always count on me. Would you be willing to do something for me first? I need to fold this basket of clothes. I could use some help. Are you willing to help me?" As the caregiver begins to fold the clothes, she can encourage the loved one to help.

"What color is that shirt you are folding?" That is a great conversation starter. Follow that conversation with questions about shirts or color or proper folding or whatever eases the situation. Soon, the individual has forgotten the desire to go home and is engrossed in folding the clothes.

However, and this is the difficult part, this same scenario will play out repeatedly. Don't think you have put an end to this desire. They will ask again, and that "again" may be in just a few moments. However, there is good news. What worked the first time to distract them will most likely work the second time. As they don't remember making the same request earlier, they will not remember the tactic you used to divert their attention.

However, there are times with the loved one will become agitated no matter what technique we employ.

"You are always keeping secrets from me. Why do you do that?"

"Oh, Momma, I am so sorry. I didn't mean to keep a secret. I have been so busy; I guess I forgot. I would never want to keep secrets from you. Can you do me a favor? Could you possibly help me organize the snacks in this cabinet? I need to see if you are out of crackers. I sure could use your help?"

Momma says, "Sure, we can do that."

This response addresses the issue, but it also changes the subject. It is evident Momma was about to get agitated. This agitation was not going to lead to anything productive, so (as Barney Fife on The Andy Griffith Show use to say), we need to, "Nip it in the bud". Stop the agitation EVERYTIME. Even if Momma is completely wrong, and you are completely correct, you need to give in! You will not convince her of anything other than what she presently believes.

A word of caution: *Don't use diversion therapy when you can actually offer a real solution.*

"I want a snack, now!" While you may be buried in work to complete, it is better to stop and get them a snack than to divert their attention. It is actually less work for you and a better ending for them. So, give consideration to opportunities to accommodate rather than divert. Diversion Therapy and Therapeutic Fibbing are two of your new best friends. Add them to your gift list this Christmas!

Smile #14

What do you call it when a dinosaur crashes his car?

Answer – Tyrannosaurus Wrecks

Sometimes, you've just got to laugh!

# YOUR HUSBAND DIED IN 1985!

I will need to take a deep breath before writing this section.  This is one of those pieces of education that should be mandatory education for anyone working in a situation as a caregiver.  It is so important!

**Never remind an individual with dementia that a loved one has died!**

Did you get that?  Just in case, let me say it another way.

**Reminding your loved one that someone died years ago is just going to bring grief!  DO NOT DO IT!**

My 15 ½ year old miniature dachshund died recently.  Grief stinks!  There are days I do well, and there are days I want to stick my head between the mattress and box springs and camp out for a while.  I often find myself intentionally changing my train of thought in order to avoid sadness I do not want to experience.

When we have dementia, emotions are heightened.  Think of the emotions as being on steroids!  They are in overdrive.  With that knowledge on board, it is easy to understand why you would not want someone reliving the death of a loved one.  Let's role play this scenario.

"John, where is your Daddy?"

"Oh, Momma", John says.  "Daddy died in 1985.  You remember.  We all came home for the funeral."

Tearfully, Mom replies, "He is dead? When did he die? I don't remember that. I can't believe he is dead. Oh my goodness. What am I going to do without him?"

John has just brought his mother to a state of panic, sadness, grief, confusion, and a few other emotions for which we may not even be aware. What if the conversation had looked like this?

"John, where is your Daddy?"

"That's a good question Momma. Last time I saw Daddy he was fishing. You know how he likes to fish. Probably having a great time, too!"

"That man sure does like to fish."

"Hey, Mom. Why don't we go for a walk and see the flowers?"

Notice how John answered the question. He didn't give her any bad news. He didn't ignore her question. Most importantly, though, he changed the subject and kept his Momma happy. This brings me to my explanation of "therapeutic fibbing".

Therapeutic fibbing is one of the best friends a caregiver can ever have. It is a talent that must be honed and sharpened. If you have a problem fibbing to your loved one, then you need to do one of two things. One – you need to figure out ways to tell the story without actually fibbing. Or, Two- get over it! I recommend you get over it. If there is one thing of which I am sure, God does not want His children with dementia upset. They have enough to deal with. Keeping them happy by using therapeutic fibbing is a favor to them. It harms no one.

# MORE ON THERAPEUTIC FIBBING

While I will be the first to remind you  The Ten Commandments advise us "You shall not bear false witness against your neighbor" (Exodus 20:16), I might also be the first to remind you of The Golden Rule.   Let's read Luke 6:31 (New International Version), "Do to others as you would have them do to you."  So what does this theology lesson have to do with dementia?

Sometimes it is loving to fib.  We all know the stories of the proper answer to "Honey, do I look fat?"  Of course, you would never say, "Yep, you look like a pig.  What has happened to you?"  That is the kind of answer that will make your life miserable, AND it should make your life miserable.  Instead, we diplomatically might answer that same question with, "Honey, you are so beautiful.  How could you think you look fat?"

Similarly, we should also be diplomatic with our loved ones with dementia.  We should even be willing to fib, if necessary.  This may be a difficult concept, but it is a necessary part of a healthy relationship with someone who has dementia.

I believe one of the best ways to make a point is with an illustration.  When my brother-in-law, Henry, was dying I was careful of the information I shared with Momma.

Momma and I have had several conversations about Henry.

"What is happening to Henry?" Momma asked.

"Well, Momma, Henry's body is dying. He is not doing well at all."

"What is causing this to happen?"

"I wish I could explain all of that, but I don't understand it myself. I know the doctors have called in Hospice, and they are offering a ton of help to Sissy while she cares for him."

Momma asked, "Is there anything I can do to help them?"

"Momma, we all need to be praying for one another. That's all any of us can do."

As you noticed, I did not go into detail regarding what was happening with Henry. I had a fairly good understanding of what was happening, but that knowledge did not bring me any comfort. Similarly, the knowledge would not bring Momma comfort, either.

The information in the brain of an individual with dementia often is confused. Picture all the new information entering a blender and being swirled around. Taking that new information and forming a logical story would be difficult. That is much the experience of someone with dementia. They have bits and pieces of information. Combining those bits and pieces into a sensible arrangement is impossible. Often the result is damaging, disturbing, upsetting, and can even cause emotional and physical pain.

In the example above, I did not tell a falsehood to my mother. However, and I don't hesitate saying this, I would do so if it kept my mother from being upset. If there is one thing I know for sure, it is this.

(It is also the one thing I hope you learn and understand thoroughly.) When my mother is upset, I can see her symptoms of dementia more clearly than at times when she is calm. These symptoms become more exacerbated, and I must spend more time trying to comfort her. It is not a good situation for either my Momma or myself. Therefore, I do whatever is necessary to keep peace and harmony flooding through my Momma's life and her mind.

Can we go back to our theology lesson for one final thought? The scripture reads, "You shall not bear false witness against your neighbor" (Exodus 20:16). Let's think about that phrase "against your neighbor". If you are lying in order to hurt someone in any way, it is wrong. There is never an exception to that rule. However, when we are using therapeutic fibbing to care for a loved one with dementia, we are not doing so in order to harm them in any way. We are not "against" them. We are "for" them in every way possible, and this is just one of the tools needed to make their life a better life. I hope that makes you feel better.

Smile #15

While working with my seniors doing music therapy, I took a singing break and asked each choir member to tell about their first job. Surprisingly, about six of my ten women worked in a dime store, and five of those six worked the candy counter! This made me wonder about the validity of their stories, but anyway. However, it was the response of one participant, who is more than a little bit deaf, which made me laugh. "So, what was your first job?" I asked. His response was so impressive that I responded with a common response in our world today. I said, "Well, Shut Up!" Now that did not mean I expected him to be quiet. Quite the opposite. I was really wanting him to tell me more. He, unfortunately, did not understand. He said, "Well, "I'll shut up and you can tell my bleepity bleep story!" Of course, he didn't say "bleepity bleep". His words were a little more colorful, if you catch my drift. Oh well. You can't win all the time.

Sometimes, you've just got to laugh!

# WHO ARE **YOU**?

As dementia progresses, our loved ones begin to forget faces. Let's tackle this sad issue together.

As the brain is being destroyed by Alzheimer's type dementia, the most recent memories are those which are lost first. Thus, your mother will forget her great grandchildren before forgetting her grandchildren. The memories will continue to fade in the reverse order in which they occurred. Therefore, the next generation to be lost to them would be their grandchildren, then their children, their spouse, and friends are lost depending upon what point the friend entered their life.

This is very hard with which to cope. I am blessed and thankful that Momma still knows me. I dread the day that is no longer true. However, I hope I will pull out this book and review the facts. These facts will help me to understand the situation, and I hope they will help you, also.

As the memories are lost, the loved one will most likely never forget their parents. The reason is simple. Their parents existed BEFORE they did. They hold memories of their parents all throughout their brain. That would also explain why so many people want to "go home to Momma". That is what they remember, and it is the time and space in which their brain is living. Pay attention to what your loved one talks about. This will help you understand "when" and "where" they are currently living. You may see the year as 2013, but they may be living in 1958. Understanding this will help you communicate regarding events that might be appropriate for 1958.

When you arrive to visit your parent, and they no longer recognize you as their child, your reaction might be, "Mom, it's me, Suzie. I'm your second daughter."

This news is very disturbing to Mom. In her mind, she is not old enough to have children, she doesn't know who you are, and she is not happy to hear something so confusing. "I don't have a daughter! I don't know who you are, so you can just leave. Help! Get this person away from me!" Your heart is breaking, your parent is agitated, and the entire situation could have been avoided.

Instead of introducing yourself as the daughter, it is better to say, "Mary, hi. It's Suzie. It's good to see you." Now Mary is approached in a way that is less stressful. The tension is absent from this scene, and Mary is able to communicate. Mary might respond with, "I knew someone named Suzie. She had curls and blond hair that looked sort of like yours." As you allow Mom to follow her own train of thought, she is more likely to have a lucid moment and connect the name "Suzie" to her own daughter. She may even say, "Hi, Suzie. How is Momma's sweet girl doing?" This is the same Mother who was adamant she did not have a daughter. These moments are fleeting, but they do occur. Enjoy them while you can.

Always approach your loved one in a way that is beneficial to everyone involved. They cannot be expected to remember events that, in their mind, have not yet happened. Stay with them in the time and place in which you find them. THEY CANNOT ENTER YOUR WORLD, BUT YOU CAN ENTER THEIR WORLD.

Relationships make our life fulfilling. Without relationships, we are solitary people who are lonely, sad, and ineffective. Relationships make us vibrant, happy, and productive. Strive to maintain the relationship you have with your loved one. When that relationship changes because of the ravages of the disease, YOU are the one to adjust. Your loved one is worth the effort necessary for you to make this adjustment. You will be glad you did!

# WHAT HAPPENS TO VISION?

There are many things that we take for granted. One of those things would be our vision. I recently had the privilege of presenting information about dementia to the folks at The National Federation of The Blind. I had the best time! They are people who do not take things for granted. I left there with a renewed desire to be aware of my blessings. Vision is one of those blessings.

As we age, we expect our vision to decrease. It is not uncommon for our elderly loved ones to see changes in their prescription, develop cataracts or glaucoma, or even have macular degeneration. Another common change is our peripheral vision.

While gazing straight ahead, extend your arms to the side and back until you cannot see them. Now begin slowly moving your arms inward, and stop at the point in which you can see your hands and arms while still looking straight ahead. Your ability to see your hands and arms, while gazing ahead, is your peripheral vision. A 20 year old person has a greater field of peripheral vision than a 70 year old person.

Dementia decreases peripheral vision dramatically. That peripheral vision is not just the ability to see left to right without moving the head. It is the ability to see top to bottom, also. Most of us can look straight ahead and still see the floor and maybe the ceiling. If you are of an advanced age, this may not be the case. If you have dementia, this most likely is not possible. The disease causing the dementia is deteriorating the occipital lobe of the brain. The vision is being affected dramatically.

So, how does this decrease in peripheral vision change life? Let me give you a few examples. As you are walking from point A to point B, you can see the folks coming toward you. If your peripheral vision is impaired, you cannot do this. The people will continue to approach, and you may become frightened when they arrive.

Consider the loss of peripheral vision from the top of the field of vision to the bottom of the field vision while climbing stairs. Imagine not being able to discern where the next step is located, how far away it is, and where to put the foot for a safe landing.

Now, take this decreased peripheral vision and add glaucoma. Glaucoma is a condition that leads to damage to the optic nerve. This nerve is important because it carries information from the eye to the brain. One of the common symptoms of glaucoma is cloudy vision. People also report rainbow-like halos which appear around lights. Now we have a disease of the eye complicated by a disease of the brain.

Other folks suffer with macular degeneration while also living with dementia. Macular Degeneration is a loss of vision in the center field of vision. Pair this with a loss of peripheral vision (left to right and top to bottom), and you can certainly understand how pairing these two conditions can cause a large problem in vision.

Let's touch on cataracts. A cataract is a clouding of the lens of the eye which reduces the passage of light. Most of us know someone with one of these common problems of the eye, and many people have more than one of these diseases. It is important to be aware of their diagnosis and match that with their capabilities.

As the dementia progresses, the vision is reduced to binocular vision. Pretend you have a pair of binoculars held to your eyes. With the binoculars, you have zero ability to see left to right. This is similar to the field of vision in someone whose dementia has advanced. Lastly, the vision decreases to monocular vision. There is only a limited amount of vision in one eye.

Bundle all these conditions and try to go about the activities of daily living. Grasping a fork, buttoning a shirt, and recognizing a face all become challenges for someone with dementia.

While the occipital lobe is being ravaged by disease, the cerebrum, which is the largest part of the brain, is also under attack. In regards to vision, the cerebrum is responsible for spatial relations. In other words, when reaching for a fork, the brain tells the hand exactly where the fork is located. There is an understanding of how far the arm needs to extend, how many inches away the fork is from the fingers, and how tight the grasp should be to hold the fork. When the cerebrum is damaged, this becomes a problem. This gives an understanding of why dressing, feeding, walking, and many more activities become a problem.

My brain is really tired, and I think I need a

break and a healthy snack. Some watermelon is in my future. Did you know eating right and exercising reduces your chances of Alzheimer's by 50%? It is true. Trash all the junk in your cabinets and add healthy fruits, nuts and seeds to your snack list.

Smile #16
Why do milking stools only have three legs?
Answer – Because the cow has the udder
Sometimes, you've just got to laugh.

# LOSS OF THE SENSE OF SMELL

There are many jokes that can be made about "smell", so I couldn't resist the urge.

Smile #17

An elderly woman went to the doctor's office for a check up. The doctor asked if she had any problems. The woman said that she had a terrible problem with constant passing of gas. However, the incidents were silent and didn't smell. In fact, she announced, she had passed gas at least 10 times since she had been in the office. Since they were silent and didn't smell, no one would have known.

The doctor listened to her story and then gave her a prescription for some pills. He told her to take these pills for a week and come back to see him. One week later the elderly woman returned to the doctor's office and complained, "I don't know what you did, but those pills have caused my wind to smell awful! They are still silent, but boy do they stink!"

The doctor replied, "Good, now that your sinuses are cleared up we will work on improving your hearing!" (author unknown)

Sometimes, you've just got to laugh!

The sense of smell is extremely important for healthy and safe living. We have five protective smells that are lost when dementia is present.

1.   The smell of smoke  -  Obviously, this could be a problem.  If you don't smell the smoke, you might stay in a burning home.

2.   The smell of gas and chemicals -   Let's assume a cup of Clorox has been placed on the washer to be used in the next load.  Grandmother walks by and sees a cup of liquid.  She is thirsty, and she drinks the Clorox.  Her sense of smell is gone, and her nose does not detect the offensive odor of Clorox before it enters her mouth.

3.   The smell of spoiled food -   It is not uncommon to find spoiled food in the refrigerator of an elderly person.  Many folks never think to remove old and outdated food, and they, therefore, consume the food.  When the food is being placed in the mouth, the nose does not detect that it is spoiled.

4.   The smell of body odor -  Senior citizens are prone to have a certain body odor.  This is due, in large part, to their lack of ability to smell themselves.

5.   Lastly, the smell of urine and feces -  This can be quite a problem.

Smell is important for our health and safety.  Be aware of the limitations your loved one may be experiencing.

# WHY THE BRA IS ON BACKWARDS

Do you remember the show "Golden Girls"? Sophia, the older of the ladies, would say, "Picture it. Sicily, 1928." And then she would tell a story.

Well, picture it. You arrive at your mother's home and discover she is dressed in two pairs of pants, and her bra is on the outside of her shirt. You are shocked! Your first impulse is to either ask her why she is dressed this way, or perhaps you might try to assist her in changing clothes.

Don't do either of these things. As far as your mother is concerned, she looks perfectly dressed, and she doesn't need you, or anyone else, changing her look. Instead, act as if she were dressed normally. That is a tall order, for sure, but it is necessary. After you have been visiting for a few minutes, you might want to have this conversation.

"Mom, I have been wondering if you might want to try on that pretty pink shirt I purchased last week."

"I didn't know you bought me a new shirt. Where is it?"

"Well, Mom, I believe it is in your closet. Let's go take a look. I need to know if it fits. If it does, we can get you some more new clothes. Let's check it out."

Mom, hopefully, agrees to explore this possibility of a new pink shirt she has forgotten about. Upon finding the shirt, discuss how pretty you think the shirt is and how it is just the right color for her skin tone. You might want to hold it up to your face to discuss how it would look on you. Just extend the conversation for a few minutes. Then try this.

"Mom, let's see how this shirt looks on you. What do you think?"

When Mom agrees to try on the shirt, you have successfully removed the offending items she was wearing, and you can now help her dress appropriately.

However, Mom still has on those two pairs of pants. It is not uncommon to see older folks wear two pairs of pants. They get cold, and two pairs of pants are great to help them stay warm. If those two pairs of pants are not unsightly, just leave them alone. What is more important in this situation? Is it more important your loved one be comfortable or pretty? Who is most worried about them being pretty? The answer to the last question is YOU. Remember, your loved one was totally content with the clothes they had on before you ever arrived.

If you have children, you can totally relate to this scene. Remember the first time your two year old dressed himself? Chances are the outcome was not exactly the look that would have landed him on the cover of GQ! However, in order not to dash his "creative spirit", you smiled and let him go as dressed. Try to use this same approach with your loved one. They are not dressed inappropriately in an attempt to embarrass you. They are not dressed inappropriately in an attempt to frustrate you. They absolutely are not aware the clothing they have on looks silly or inappropriate.

I have one last tip for your tool chest of options. If your loved one is wearing several pieces of clothing, you could always ask what size the top piece might be. Try as you may, you cannot discern that size without them taking that piece of clothing off. Once they have, use your diversion therapy techniques to help them forget they were ever wearing that article of clothing to begin with.

Helping our loved ones most always requires a certain amount of creativity on our part. It is better for us to be creative than to risk hurting their feelings. Their life is hard enough. They don't need any extra stress!

Smile #18
What washes up on tiny beaches?
Answer – Micro-waves!
Sometimes, you've just got to laugh!

# SOMEBODY NEEDS A BATH

Bathing is such a hot topic with some families. Most of us are accustomed to bathing every night or every morning. Some of us do both! The thoughts of our loved one bathing only once or twice a week is more than we can handle.

As we age, our skin becomes fragile and sensitive. Bathing can actually be painful to an elderly person. The fat pads between the skin and bone are much thinner, the skin itself is thin, and the nerve endings are more sensitive to touch. Therefore, rubbing the skin with a washcloth can actually be painful. Standing under the shower can bring about an entirely different set of problems. Let's think about that.

I totally enjoy standing under a hard stream of hot water until the hot water is totally gone. I love to feel it beat on my head as it massages my scalp. My mother, on the other hand, may not find this process to be so wonderful.

Let us remember a few important details about bathing. Bathing requires us to become naked. When helping your loved one, you are asking them to remove all their clothing in front of you or a caregiver! They are thinking, "I am not getting naked in front of these people. I don't even know them." Often times a caregiver will encourage a resident or loved one to disrobe in order to shower. The resident refuses, and the caregiver exacerbates the problem by asking a second caregiver to come into the bathroom to assist. Now we have a resident being asked to become totally naked in front of TWO strangers. This is not a good situation, and it will not turn out well.

Let's try this approach, instead. When asking someone to disrobe, offer them a beach towel or bathrobe with which to cover themselves. If that does not work, tell them you will hold the beach towel in front of them while they remove their clothing one piece at a time. Be sure to let them know you will be turning your head away while they undress. If they insist on wearing their underclothes, go with it!

Before they enter the shower or tub, make sure you have already started the water to the correct temperature - not too hot and not too cold. Make sure you are using a shower seat. Always have your loved one bathe or shower from the shower seat. It is safer for them and easier for you. Place the shower seat in the proper position for their comfort.

Let me recommend another wonderful addition to the bathing apparatus. Bathing is easier when you have a handheld shower head. This allows for several very important features. I will tell you more in a moment, but let's get that loved one IN the shower first.

Since some folks may not desire to enter the shower or tub at all, you need to have a few tricks up your sleeve to help make the transition easier. First of all, turn the water off. Allow them to be seated on the shower seat, totally covered for modesty, and talk with them. There is no need to rush. Even if you have a thousand things on your agenda for the day, rushing your loved one with dementia will NEVER speed any process. After they have relaxed a bit while seated on the shower seat, position the handheld showerhead at their feet. Announce that you are going to turn the water on very gently for the purpose of washing their feet.

This is where the importance of a handheld showerhead comes into play. When we use a showerhead that is mounted high, the water comes from above and falls on us. As mentioned earlier, this may be painful for our seniors who have thin skin. It also may be frightening. Look at it from their prospective. They are seated comfortably and, all of a sudden, water painfully covers their body. From where did the water come? How did it get in the shower? What can be done to stop it? It is not uncommon to hear them shout, "How do I get out of here? HELP!"

Always announce what movement you are planning to make. "Mrs. Smith, I am going to turn the water on. It will come out this end and land on your feet. Is it OK if I wash your toes?" Most likely, Mrs. Smith will agree. If she does not, be careful not to push the situation. A good response if she is not cooperative is, "Maybe I will turn the water on and wash this side of the shower stall. It looks a bit dirty. Don't you think that is a good idea?" Once Mrs. Smith sees the water coming out of the showerhead, feels its run on the soles of her feet, she is more likely to respond positively to the idea of having her toes and feet washed. REMINDER – Do not scrub! The skin is sensitive.

Once Mrs. Smith has agreed to have her feet washed, begin asking permission to work your way up her legs. Skip over to her hands and arms, then her neck and back. Next you need to be most cautious while attempting to wash the genitalia. Mrs. Smith is very self-conscious. She has left her panties in place, and you need to respect her right to do so. You might give her a wet washcloth and suggest she wash beneath her panties. This gives her a sense of privacy, and also allows for the mission to be accomplished. You can rinse this area through the panties with no difficulty.

Once Mrs. Smith has completed the washing process, proceed with the drying process in much the same way. Allow Mrs. Smith to have another dry beach towel with which to cover, or turn your gaze to allow for some privacy. It is very possible to dress an individual in clean underclothes while they hold a beach towel between you and them.

The point to remember is this. Treat people kindly. Don't assume what you want is what is best for them. Don't assume what you want is necessary for them. Don't assume what you understand to be true is how they see a situation. Remember these words - "I'M ENTERING THEIR WORLD" - and you will be an excellent caregiver.

Now that we have finished bathing, it is time for a CLEAN joke – pun intented! This story actually happened to a friend of mine.

Smile #19
Dad had suffered with dementia for many years. Upon a visit by his son and family, the

daughter-in-law reminded the dad to wait for his son to get to the room before he proceeded with taking a shower. This man had a tendency to strip down and strut around (so to speak) in all of his natural beauty! "You just wait until your son gets here, and he will help you bathe." Dad was not interested in this piece of advice. He proceeded to shower and towel off. Having completed this task, Dad walked, stark naked, into the living room with a washcloth strategically placed over his ---CHEST! He knew he needed to cover up, so he did just that. The girls in the room were shocked, of course. However, Dad was totally confident in his decision to be modest!

Sometimes, you've just got to laugh!

# HALLUCINATIONS CAN BE INTERESTING

Have you ever been around someone who was hallucinating? These situations can be funny, and they can be scary. There is no way to predict which direction these hallucinations will go. It is important to know why they happen and how to respond (or how NOT to respond) to them.

Why do people with dementia hallucinate? When there is damage to the frontal cortex and prefrontal cortex (think about your forehead), hallucinations can occur. The brain begins to make up stories. These stories are referred to as "confabulation". In addition to the frontal cortex being damaged, the sensory strip is damaged as well as the visual center. This would explain why people actually see events or people that no one else is seeing.

If your loved one is experiencing hallucinations, go with the story. Do not attempt to stop the hallucination unless the process has the potential to be harmful in some way. Also, never tell the individual they are not seeing what they claim to be seeing. They actually are experiencing life just as they are explaining it to you. The brain makes up stories. These stories, or events, are totally real. Trying to convince someone they are NOT seeing what they are sure they are seeing is useless. It is detrimental to the health of the situation and the health of the individual. You will only frustrate and anger them. Do not argue with them. Go with the flow. Enter their world.

Hallucinations are common in Lewy Body Disease dementia. Most often these hallucinations are about animals, children, and sex. I had a client who was extremely deaf, but she was insistent she could hear the couple next door having sex. She even called the police, repeatedly, regarding this event. It was extremely frightening for her, and it was very annoying for her family. Telling her the event was not taking place was useless. She knew what she heard, and she absolutely did not want anyone telling her otherwise. As a result, I would listen to her stories, and then I would try to divert her attention to another subject.

Another reason an individual might hallucinate would be a side effect of a medication. If hallucinations begin, investigate whether there has been a change in medication. The addition of a new drug or an increase in an existing drug can be the reason an individual may hallucinate. Drug abuse or misuse can lead to hallucinations.

Hallucinations can also be the body's way of letting you know something is wrong. The individual could have an infection, such as a urinary tract infection, a bladder infection, be in pain, be constipated, need to urinate, have skin breakdown, or even be dehydrated. Anytime behavior changes, investigate the reason for the change. Do not automatically resort to drugs to change the behavior.

Why not automatically turn to medications to

help with behaviors?  The drugs used would likely be anti-psychotic type drugs.  These drugs have been shown to lead to an increase in stroke and death.  It is better to work with behavior and environmental changes to bring about the desired results.  Once you have determined the presence or lack of physical pain or discomfort as the source of the hallucination, you should look at the environment.  Is the room crowded?  Is it noisy?  Are there flashing lights?  Is someone arguing with the individual hallucinating?  Is there a particular person that seems to make the hallucinations occur more frequently?  Being observant of the individual, their surroundings, and their reactions is key to helping manage hallucinations without medication.

One last thought.  Never use restraints.  Restraints would include any device that confines or restricts the movement or activity of an individual.  The use of restraints brings about a loss of dignity and freedom.  They have also been shown to result in increased falls, incontinence and, pressure ulcerations.


Smile #20

While singing gospel songs at an assisted living, the duet was happy to lead the residents in a rousing rendition of "I Saw the Light".  Much to the shock of everyone in the room, a resident came walking into the room, singing along loudly, stark naked!  The guitarist commented, "I saw the light, and I saw the moon."  Whenever he sings that song, he has this image of a naked man singing along while walking through the room.

Sometimes, you've just got to laugh!

# NURTURING THERAPY

I remember the days when Momma would allow me to rest my head in her lap while she rubbed my ears. Other times, she would scratch my head. I can also recall coming home from school and smelling supper in the oven. These are all forms of nurturing therapy.

Recently, I had abdominal surgery. My mother, who has Alzheimer's, very much wanted to help care for me after surgery. However, Momma's abilities to help were limited. Well, so I thought. On the way home from surgery, it seemed my husband hit every bump in the road. Of course, this is not true, but my abdomen thought otherwise. I began to cry and said, "Michael, I need my Momma. Please go by and pick her up." Although I was still somewhat under the influence of some really good drugs at the time, Michael honored my request.

Upon arriving home, Momma positioned me comfortably on the sofa and proceeded to care for me. What I wanted, more than anything, was to lay my head in her lap. I asked if I could do this, and she was happy to offer her lap for my comfort. She scratched my head, played with my hair, massaged my ears, and just made me feel good. Then, being the thoughtful daughter I am, I turned around and put my feet in her lap and let her continue this process! Aren't I sweet?

This type of care is called "nurturing therapy". It is therapy that brings us back to a place and time that felt good. These memories bring us peace, joy, smiles, comfort, and a host of other really good emotions. For some people, nurturing therapy may include a baby doll. While some people find it embarrassing for their loved one to carry a doll around, they need to understand our loved ones have often gone back in time to the point where they were parenting a small child or a baby. Holding this baby doll might spark those memories. They find great comfort in stroking the doll, changing the clothes, putting the doll down for a nap, and – believe it or not – remembering to retrieve the doll after the nap. These are the same people who cannot tell you they need to use the bathroom, but they will amazingly remember to get a doll out of a crib after a nap! If this type of therapy is enjoyable for your loved one, please do not stop the process. It is healthy!

I am sure you have experienced the pleasure of stroking the back of a sweet dog or cat. This is nurturing therapy, also. It calms the nerves and lowers the blood pressure. It brings a sense of relaxation and connection that might not otherwise exist.

In my local emergency room is a wonderful nurse who understands nurturing therapy. When she is working with an individual in the advanced stages of dementia, she will roll up a warmed towel and ask the individual to hold the towel close to their chest as a favor to her. "I am really busy, and I was hoping you would hold this for me." She never refers to it as a towel. She merely asks for assistance. This appeals to the individual's desire to be needed, and it allows them to nurture the "baby" they are holding. It calms the individuals, and this nurse can get her work accomplished with less resistance.

My grandmother, Bessie, had a doll she named Griz Maliz. No one knew where the name came from, but Grandma enjoyed her doll. Other people might enjoy a stuffed animal. The point is simple. If it makes your loved one happy, go with it. Often we spend too much time trying to get people to do or act or be a certain way. Learning to "go with the flow" early in life will make us better caregivers later in life. Remember, ENTER THEIR WORLD!

# MUSIC THERAPY –
## OH HOW I LOVE **IT**!

Without a doubt, music therapy is the favorite part of my professional life. I have the extreme honor and blessing to be a music therapy coach. I take music therapy into facilities, group homes, adult day cares, or individual homes. Through these experiences, I have witnessed some extraordinary events take place.

Let's talk about the mechanics of the brain again for a moment. The part of the brain that holds music, prayer, poetry, and art are least affected by dementia. I find this amazing. Further, the part of the brain that holds speech is not the same part of the brain that holds music. Let me explain.

Your temporal lobe is the area around your ears. So your right temporal lobe is around your right ear. This right lobe holds rhythm. Rhythm remains in dementia patients. You can remember this with the letter "R". Remember the early days of "Sesame Street" on television and their 'letter of the day'? Well, today's letter is "The Letter R". "R" stands for right, rhythm and remains. The "right" side of the brain holds "rhythm" that "remains" despite the disease in the brain.

Tomorrow's letter of the day will be "L". The left temporal lobe is the area around your left ear. It holds language. Language is lost with this brain disease. So, "L" stands for left, language, lost. The "left" side of the brain holds "language that is lost" due to the disease in the brain.

Understanding that language and rhythm are housed in two different parts of the brain will explain why an individual who stutters can sing without any problem. The stuttering is part of language that is found in the left temporal lobe. The ability to sing is part of rhythm that resides in the right temporal lobe.

"R" stands for right, rhythm and remains.

"L" stands for left, language, and lost.

I would like to share a few specific stories from my music therapy experiences. I have the privilege of directing seven choirs, and one is at the assisted living home where my mother lives. Most of my participants have some level of cognitive disability.

One day I invited a lady to join choir practice. She spent her days curled up in her wheelchair. The employees informed me of her inability to talk, but I was not worried. I wheeled her into practice. She listened, but she showed little sign of interest. The next week, I repeated the process. At that time, we were practicing Christmas music for our upcoming Christmas show. After just a few songs, I heard this high pitch voice that I did not recognize. It was this lady, and she was singing!

I was so excited. It would have been a totally wonderful experience, except she wasn't singing the song we were singing. Oh well, just a minor detail. I placed myself directly in front of her, took her hands in mine, and sang to her. I sang while looking in her eyes and smiling. Much to my happiness, she started singing the same song. That song was "Away in a Manger". When the choir finished singing, she continued. She sang the entire second verse to this Carol as a solo. My pianist and I were shocked. It was at that moment I knew we would have her do this at the Christmas show.

As the night approached, I positioned this lovely lady in the front row of the choir. Suddenly, she disappeared. Her family decided she needed to visit the bathroom before the performance. I said to them, "Please bring her back quickly. She is singing a solo." They replied, "Granny doesn't even speak. There is no way she is going to sing a solo." Being the Southerner I am, I responded, "Hide and watch!" Well, sing a solo she did! She sang the second verse to "Away in a Manger" with all the gusto you can imagine. When she finished she said, "AMEN!" Upon observing the audience, I discovered there wasn't a dry eye in the house. It was an absolutely wonderful experience.

Later, this same lady was taken to the emergency room for treatment to her face. She had fallen out of her wheelchair, and her face had received damage from the fall. She needed stitches. She was absolutely sure this doctor was not getting anywhere near her with the needle and proceeded to curse this doctor. Her daughter-in-law, aware of this lady's recent solo at Christmas, began to sing "Let It Snow". My friend joined her daughter-in-law in singing, stopped cursing, sat still, and the doctor took care of business. However, and this is an important part of the story, she cursed her family the entire way home! As I have told you many times, sometimes, you just have to laugh!

I have also watched Parkinson's patients become still and hands that normally shake violently start swaying at the sound of music. The head stops shaking, the rhythm takes over, and the individual joins the song. Music is amazing.

I am sure you can remember a time in life when you were down in the dumps, then you heard a song on the radio. Maybe that song reminded you of your first love, or a vacation, or your child, or whatever. It transported you from the present day and time to another day and time. Music is healing. Music is soothing. Music is a gift from God. I am so glad it remains no matter the devastation of the disease.

While not necessarily "music", sayings from our past that are rhythmic are processed in our brains much the same way as music. For example, if I were to say, "A stitch in time" you might respond with "saves nine". "Jack and Jill" might elicit "went up the hill". These sayings are rhythmic and spark the right side of the brain to recall the words needed to finish the rhyme.

Another type of recall in the right side of the brain is automatic speech. These are phrases we have heard that are not necessarily rhythmic, but they bring a response automatically. Here are a few examples. See how good you are at completing the phrase.

Eat like a _____.
All you need is _____.
Never judge a book _____.
If life deals you lemons, _____.

2, 4, 6, 8, who do we _____.
Face that only a mother _____.
Honor thy father _____.
It isn't nice to fool _____.
Kid tested, mother _____.
A fool and his money _____.
Love of money is the _____.
Money doesn't grow _____.
Ask a silly question and you'll get _____.

Answers: horse, love, by its cover, make lemonade, appreciate, could love, and mother, mother nature, approved, are soon parted, root of all evil, on trees, a silly answer

Smile #21
(Sing this to the tune of "Three Blind Mice")
Three decrepit rodents, three decrepit rodents,

Observe how they motivated, observe how they motivated

They all motivated after the agricultural executive's spouse

Who amputated their posterior with a carving utensil

Have you ever observed such a phenomenon in your existence?

As three decrepit rodents!

You've just got to laugh!

(Original version written by Thomas Ravenscroft in 1609.)

# MAKE YOUR HOME SAFE

Making the home of your loved one safe is important whether they have dementia or not. Here are a few suggestions.

1.  No throw rugs. They can easily cause an individual to fall.

2. If your loved one is in a wheelchair, place pictures and artwork at eye level. Remove pictures of people from their recent past and replace with pictures from the long ago past.

3. Remove clutter. Be prepared, however, this cleaning up process may be met with strong resistance. Be respectful of the individual's desire to keep items. However, these items need to be out of traffic patterns.

4. Remove old and outdated foods from cupboards and refrigerators. This is a continual process.

5. Remove knives and sharp items.

6. Assign two cabinets to hold items most often used or eaten.

7. Remove the doors from those two cabinets. This will allow ease of access and reduce the time spent searching for items.

8. Put safety locks on remaining cabinets or leave them empty. Make sure medicines are stored in a safe place.

9. Install a raised toilet seat.

10. Install a shower seat

11. Install a grab bar in the shower

12. Make sure each room has ease of access for a wheelchair bound individual.

13. Install a handheld shower head.

14. Label drawers in the kitchen and the bedroom. Maintaining continuity in where items are stored is always helpful.

15. Remove mirrors. Seeing themselves in the mirror can be frightening as they are not aware they have aged.

16. Purchase a clock with large letters that also states the day and date.

17. Keep hazardous items (bug spray, Clorox, hair spray) out of reach.

18. Remove clothing that is no longer needed or ill-fitting.

19. Launder clothing in a mild detergent. Adding baking soda to the wash cycle can help reduce urine odors in fabric. Use about one-half cup to an average load size.

20. Arrange clothing in sets on the hanger. Hanging a shirt with a matching pair of pants will save confusion for the caregiver, and will assure your loved one's appearance is acceptable.

21. Place a clean washcloth in the shower each day. It is not unusual for someone to use the same towel and washcloth repeatedly. Avoid this issue by routinely changing out these items.

22. Place a bottle of water by your loved one's favorite chair. This will aid in keeping them hydrated.

These are just a few ideas. The more you work with your loved one, the more ideas you will acquire to make their home cozy and safe.

# IT'S ALL ABOUT THEM

"The relationship is what counts – not the outcome" is a phrase I learned from Teepa Snow (www.teepasnow.com). I have repeated that phrase to clients, and to myself, many times. It is a phrase that is appropriate whether we are living with dementia, providing care for someone with dementia, or just dealing with the human race. Relationship is the most important part of our life. I believe the ultimate relationship begins and ends with Jesus Christ. All the relationships in the middle are gifts from Him, and we are to cherish and honor those gifts.

There are times, when working with a person with dementia, you are well aware the words being said are inaccurate, not truthful, or just simply hurtful. Correcting the person is not the approach needed. In the grand scheme of things, what they are saying just doesn't matter. Remind yourself of this – They are speaking from a brain that is severely damaged. You are listening from a brain that is healthy. Which brain should do the "giving in" in this situation?

It is often difficult to answer the same question repeatedly, but it is more difficult for them to realize they never seem to have answers to life's questions. Try to look at life from the perspective with which your loved one is living. It will help you see things differently.

I have recently begun to notice a change in Momma. This change is not harming Momma, nor is it upsetting to her. She seems to need extra attention. She thrives on the being the center of attention, and she especially likes it when I pamper and pet her. So I seek opportunities to involve her in my everyday life.

Recently, I arrived at Momma's apartment and announced we were going to change the sheets on her bed. Together we worked to accomplish this. I then suggested she go home with me and help change the bed linens on both beds in my home. She was happy to help. I was happy to have the extra hands at work. Then Momma stretched out across the freshly made bedspread, enjoyed the sun coming in on her face, and said, "Read me the blogs you have recently written." (Yes, she has learned what a blog is!) After a few minutes, Momma dozed off, I worked on this book, and I enjoyed the moment.

The events of life are not so important. The moments are essential. It is all about relationships.

SMILE #22

The young mother was trying to potty train her little boy. She enticed him to sit on the potty, left him alone, and returned a few minutes later. She asked, "Have you used the potty yet?" "No, I can't. My bottom doesn't work because it doesn't have any batteries in it."

Sometimes, you've just got to laugh!

# WHAT CAN I DO TO PREVENT DEMENTIA?

This chapter may be the most important of this book, and it may be the most disliked as well. There are things that can be done to help prevent Alzheimer's type dementia. This is great news. The bad news is most people are not willing to take the good advice offered.

You can reduce your chances of having Alzheimer's type dementia by 50% simply by eating right and exercising. This is excellent news. However, most folks are used to eating whatever they desire, living a sedentary life, and avoiding proper vitamin and supplement nutrition. These bad decisions lead to a host of health problems.

Let's begin with the various health problems that arise from poor eating and lack of exercise. We are all familiar with high blood pressure, high cholesterol and diabetes. All of these are issues that cause concern in regards to good overall health. These same diseases increase your chances of Alzheimer's. This is startling news for many folks, but it makes sense. When the blood does not reach the brain as it should, the brain is not able to function at full capacity. Anything that slows the flow of blood to the brain is detrimental to the health of the brain.

Stressing the importance of healthy eating is a topic for which I am passionate. I have lost 100 pounds by eating healthy and exercising. I have a very real understanding of how difficult this task was to accomplish, and I live daily with the challenge to lose an additional 25 pounds. It is very difficult to achieve success in the area of eating healthy every day of my life. However, when I choose to eat foods that are preserved, artificial, sugar laden, loaded with flour, or high in fat, I always pay the price. For me, I have extreme physical symptoms within an hour of having eaten those foods. For most people, the symptoms or results of having eaten those foods do not appear for months or years. Then the body begins to speak through elevated cholesterol levels, blood pressure that is out of normal range, blood glucose levels that are dangerous, and a host of other issues. In a large majority of cases, these issues can be corrected by eating correctly and exercising. Yet, as is common with Americans today, the desire for gratification or instant happiness becomes more important than the long-term goal of good health.

Because Alzheimer's type dementia is prevalent in our world, and very present in my family history, I find it easier to stay away from those foods that are bad for me. I have made it my goal to eat a plant-based diet. I consume fruits, vegetables, whole grains, beans, nuts and seeds. While I have chosen not to eat meat or meat by-products, I am not suggesting this for everyone else. If you are comfortable eating lean meats, eggs, cheese, etc., then please do so. Just make sure you are eating plenty of plant-based foods along with the meat and meat by-products.

If food comes in a box, or bag, has colorful writing, and a list of ingredients I can't pronounce, you can feel confident that food item is not in my grocery cart. The biggest exception would be the following product.

That product is a bread called Ezekiel 4:9. It is sold in the freezer section of most grocery stores, and it has nothing artificial or preserved in its ingredients. I highly recommend you try it. My most favorite type is the cinnamon raisin. So yummy!

In addition to eating healthy, we must exercise. OK, stop snarling your nose at me. I totally understand the lack of desire to exercise. I am in that camp also. However, when I get myself off the sofa, put on my walking shoes, and trot outside, I find a release of stress and an increase in good feelings.

If the weather is too hot or too cold, there are plenty of DVD's you can purchase to exercise inside your home. I recommend Leslie Sansone's, 'Walk Away the Pounds' series. I own about ten different versions, and they are all GREAT.

Just make sure you exercise! It is too important to your health and your future for you to ignore. MOVE! MOVE! MOVE!

A recent study showed strength training to be beneficial for those who already have Alzheimer's. In a controlled study, individuals were given a cognitive assessment; half the participants did nothing to change their level of activity. The other half increased their activity to include thirty minutes of strength training twice per week. The folks who strength trained showed an increase in their scores on the cognitive assessment at the end of the trial. If exercise is good for us even while living with the disease, imagine how much healthier we are if we exercise BEFORE we get the disease.

Supplements and herbs can aid in keeping us healthy. Ginkgo Biloba is an herb that comes from one of the oldest living tree species. It contains flavonoids and terpenoids. These chemicals are believed to have antioxidant properties. It is believed to help prevent Alzheimer's. Notice, I did not say it WOULD prevent Alzheimer's. However, it is worth the chance of trying if your doctor approves.

What does antioxidant properties mean? Antioxidants are good in that they scavenge free radicals. Free radicals are bad in that they damage cells. Free radicals are believed to cause a host of problems, including heart disease, cancer, and Alzheimer's disease. Ginkgo Biloba has antioxidants that help neutralize free radicals. This prevents them from causing damage in the body. I presently am taking 120 milligrams per day, but that is my personal preference.

Ginkgo Biloba is inexpensive and available at most chain drug stores and discount stores. Be sure and check with your doctor BEFORE you add Ginkgo Biloba to your diet.

It is also believed that ibuprofen helps reduce the chances of getting Alzheimer's. A dosage of 200 milligrams per day is recommended. However, you should check with your doctor before taking ibuprofen. There are several medical conditions which prohibit the addition of ibuprofen. Be careful! Also, if you take aspirin each day, do not add ibuprofen. The combination is not good.

Fish oil is another good supplement I have added to my daily regime. My preferred source for this supplement is "OmegaPlex" by AdvoCare (go to www.advocare.com and type in Carol Howell as your distributor). Fish oil is good for your heart as well!

Vitamin B Complex is also important, and I take it as directed on the bottle. Why Vitamin B Complex? Remember, a drop in vitamin B can cause sudden onset of reversible dementia. Avoid this problem by adding vitamin B on a regular basis, but ONLY IF YOUR DOCTOR AGREES. NOTE: If you are anemic, ask your doctor about Vitamin B injections instead of supplements.

Vitamin E is another supplement recommended for good health. I take 200 international units per day. In addition, it is good to add Vitamin C at the rate of 1000 milligrams twice per day. Vitamin C aids in the absorption of Vitamin E. However, the acid in Vitamin C can be hard on the tummy. Be careful.

Now, just to cover all bases, please read the following out loud in front of a huge group of people.

I WILL NOT TAKE ANY OF THE RECOMMENDED DRUGS, SUPPLEMENTS, HERBS, OR VITAMINS WITHOUT FIRST CHECKING WITH MY PHYSICIAN. THE AUTHOR ACCEPTS NO RESPONSIBILITY FOR ME DOING OTHERWISE.

OK, now that we have the legal junk covered, let's stop for a joke.

Smile #23

Friend and author James Watkins laughed when he said,

"I think my State of Mind just seceded from the Union".

Sometimes, you've just got to laugh!

I have a trick that will help you process information more quickly. I want you to close your eyes for about ten minutes, rest your mind, relax your body, and maybe, just maybe you will doze off for a few minutes. Wake me, please, when you are ready to read again.

Ahh, do you feel all refreshed. Guess what? All the information you read just before taking that nap is more securely lodged in your brain, and will be easier for you to recall up to a week later than had you not taken the brief nap. Isn't that good news? I always knew I liked to nap, and now I have a good reason to do so.

A study done by the University of Edinburgh, in Scotland, showed these wonderful results in people who are not experiencing a cognitive decrease. Hopefully, that would be you and I. So, take the time to sleep eight full hours at night, and allow yourself the pleasure of a short break to relax your body and mind.

Another helpful thing to do is to sit with a tennis ball in your hand. Grasp the tennis ball with a firm grip. Close your eyes, relax your body, and hold onto the ball. As you begin to relax, the grip on the tennis ball will lessen and eventually you will drop the ball. When it hits the floor, the noise will awaken you. This generally takes about 10-15 minutes. Just long enough to rejuvenate the mind, body, and spirit.

# REVIEW AND STATISTICS

It has been a pleasure to spend time with you. I hope you have learned quite a bit about Alzheimer's and the various dementias. Most of all, it is my desire that you gained SMILES regarding the process of providing care for your loved one. Remember, "KNOWLEDGE brings POWER. Power brings HOPE. Hope brings SMILES. We all need more SMILES!"

Let me leave you with a few statistics and points for review.

- 3 out of 10 people get diagnosed in the early stage of their disease

- Most people have symptoms 2-5 years before they are diagnosed.

- Recognize an individual's preferences and life history. When their preferences do not match with their actions, it is often a scream for help.

- Individuals will mask symptoms at the doctor's visit because they are experiencing something different/new/special. This can actually cause the brain to fire and make the individual seem well.

- Do WITH, not TO an individual.

- Remember, we are dealing with brain failure.

- There are at least four certainties of Alzheimer's type dementia. (1) At least two parts of the brain are affected and dying. (2) It is chronic (long-lasting) and nothing can be done to stop, slow, or reverse it. (3) It can't be prevented, but we can reduce the risk. (4) It will get worse, and it is terminal.

-   Diabetics are 77% more likely to have Alzheimer's type dementia or vascular dementia.

-   4 out of 10 people in mid-stage dementia are still driving.

-   If an individual with dementia is driving and in an accident, on average, they will kill themselves and 2 other people.

-   Impulse control is gone, but impulses remain.

-   Being right doesn't always mean a good outcome!

-   Vision changes are evident. Peripheral vision is a protective vision. It allows knowledge that something or someone is approaching. Alzheimer's decreases peripheral vision.

-   Discriminating vision tells us WHAT is coming towards us. This vision is also decreased.

-   Example of lost vision – Close right eye. Look through circled fingers with left eye. Holding a pen in your right hand, try to touch something in front of you with that pen.

-   Admit when YOU are wrong. Say, "I am sorry I yelled. I am sorry. I was wrong. I am sorry. This is just HARD!"

-   Acknowledge the person first and the dementia second.

-   Each person is unique, but the disease is predictable.

- Once you have seen one person with dementia, it means you have seen ONE person with dementia. Everyone responds based on his or her own personality and history.

Lastly, don't travel the journey of dementia alone. Find a support group. The Alzheimer's Association offers support groups throughout The United States. Visit www.alz.org to find one near you.

One of the joys of my life is working one-on-one with individuals who are providing care. I am an Endorsed Life Coach with an emphasis on Music Therapy. My life coaching services are available no matter where you live. With Skype and FaceTime, we can meet in the comfort of our own homes and learn together. Visit my website at www.seniorlifejourneys.com to learn more.

Blessings and smiles on you, always.

I would like to take a moment to acknowledge the extraordinary talent and wisdom of Teepa Snow (www.teepasnow.com). Her seminars, webinars, and website have been a valuable source of knowledge for me. I have grown in my knowledge of dementia, and sharpened my skills of laughter, due – in large part – to her work. "Thank you, Teepa!"

# ABOUT THE AUTHOR

Carol Howell is a Certified Dementia Specialist and Endorsed Life Coach with an emphasis on Music Therapy. After her husband's brain injury in 1992 and her mother's diagnosis of Alzheimer's in 2006, Carol felt the need to learn about the brain. As her knowledge increased, she became more intrigued and determined to become an equipped and prepared caregiver. Her company, Senior Life Journeys, was born from this desire to learn and help others.

Carol is the author of IF MY BODY IS A TEMPLE, WHY AM I EATING DOUGHNUTS? It tells of the "amazing miracle" that helped her lose 100 pounds. The book is written with the humor and sincerity Carol is known to display in her own life.

Carol also authored LET'S TALK DEMENTIA - A Caregiver's Guide. This easy to read book is full of helpful tips for caregiving, information about dementia, and 23 SMILES that will brighten your day.

Carol resides in South Carolina with her husband, Michael, and they are the proud parents of a daughter who is a physician assistant in Florida.